A MANUAL OF
NORMAL NEONATAL CARE

A MANUAL OF
NORMAL NEONATAL CARE

second edition

N R C Roberton MA, MB, FRCP

Formerly Consultant Paediatrician,
Addenbrooke's Hospital; Director of the Regional
Neonatal Intensive Care Unit, Rosie Maternity
Hospital; Associate Lecturer in Paediatrics,
Cambridge University; Fellow of Fitzwilliam College,
Cambridge, UK

A member of the Hodder Headline Group
LONDON • SYDNEY • AUCKLAND
Co-published in the USA by Oxford University Press Inc., New York

First published in Great Britain in 1988
Second edition published in 1996 by Arnold, a member of
the Hodder Headline Group,
338 Euston Road, London NW1 3BH

Co-published in the United States of America by
Oxford University Press, Inc.,
198 Madison Avenue, New York, NY 10016
Oxford is a registered trademark of Oxford
University Press

Whilst the advice and information in this book is believed
to be true and accurate at the date of going to press,
neither the author nor the publisher can accept any legal
responsibility or liability for any errors or omissions that
may be made. In particular (but without limiting the
generality of the preceding disclaimer) every effort has
been made to check drug dosages; however it is still
possible that errors have been missed. Furthermore, dosage
schedules are constantly being revised and new side-effects
recognized. For these reasons the reader is strongly urged
to consult the drug companies' printed instructions before
administering any of the drugs recommended in this book.

British Library Cataloguing in Publication Data
A catalogue record for this book is available from the
British Library

Library of Congress Cataloging-in-Publication Data
A catalog record for this book is available from the Library
of Congress

ISBN 0 340 61375 0

Typeset in New Baskerville by Anneset,
Weston-super-Mare, Avon
Printed and bound in Hong Kong by Shiny International
Ltd.

CONTENTS

PREFACE   xiii

I INTRODUCTION   1

The normal term baby   2
Special babies   3
References   3

2 DEFINITIONS AND STATISTICS   5

Gestation   5
Birthweight   6
Birthweight for gestation   7
Embryo   10
Fetus   10
Post-conceptional age   10
Viability   10
Perinatal, neonatal, infant   12
Mortality statistics   12
Reference   15

3 THE EFFECT OF MATERNAL ILLNESS, BAD HABITS OR
  THERAPY ON THE BABY   16

Maternal illness   16
Maternal substance abuse   38
Maternal drug therapy   41
References   51
Further reading   52

4 RESUSCITATION OF THE NEWBORN   53

Causes of delayed onset of regular
  respiration   53
Physiology of asphyxia   54

Relevance of animal experiments to
clinical neonatal care 57
Assessment of the severity of asphyxia 58
Resuscitation 60
Problems with resuscitation 69
Parental involvement 72
References 72
Further reading 72

5 CARE OF THE NORMAL BABY IN THE DELIVERY SUITE 73

Temperature control 73
Cord clamping 75
Cord care 75
Labelling 76
Eye prophylaxis 76
Vitamin K 77
Bathing 78
Measurement 78
Bonding 79
References 80

6 ROUTINE POSTNATAL CARE 81

Home versus hospital 81
Admission routine 81
Rooming-in 82
Sleeping position 82
The normal neonate 82
Prevention of infection on a postnatal
ward 84
Fate of the foreskin 86
Well baby care 86

7 EXAMINATION OF THE NEWBORN 87

General principles 87
Systematic evaluation 88
The routine neonatal clinical examination
(RNCE) 106

Gestational age assessment 109
References 112
Further reading 113

8 NEONATAL BIOCHEMICAL SCREENING 114

Phenylketonuria 114
Hypothyroidism 115
Other inborn errors of amino acid
  metabolism 117
Galactosaemia 117
Cystic fibrosis 117
Other conditions 118
Clinical screening 118

9 INFANT FEEDING 119

Lactation 119
Breast milk composition 121
Volume 125
Cows' milk and cows' milk based formulae 126
Soya milks 130
Other milks 131
The breast versus bottle controversy 132
The practicalities of feeding neonates 140
Feeding problems 153
References 165
Further reading 167

10 CRITERIA FOR ADMISSION TO NEONATAL UNITS 168

Introduction 168
Risks of nosocomial infection 169
Misinterpretation of data 170
Advances in obstetric and neonatal care 171
Misuse of facilities 171
Mother–child separation 171
Conclusion 172
References 174

11   CARE OF SMALL BABIES ON A POSTNATAL WARD   175

    Organisation   175
    Criteria for admission   175
    Care of the mothers of low birthweight
      infants   176
    Staffing the PNW   176
    Routine medical care of small babies   177
    Temperature control   178
    The normal pre-term infant   180
    The normal small-for-dates baby   181
    Feeding low birthweight babies   186
    Discharging small babies   193
    Post-discharge care   193
    References   194

12   TWINS   196

    Types of twin   196
    Establishing zygosity   196
    Medical care of twins   197
    Feeding   199
    Discharging twins   201
    Well baby care   201
    Triplets and higher multiples   201
    Further reading   202

13   BIG BABIES   203

    Introduction   203
    Feeding   205
    Weight   205
    Jaundice   205
    Weaning   206
    Reference   206
    Further reading   206

14	POSTMATURE BABIES	207
	Postnatal ward care	207
15	THE INFANT OF THE DIABETIC MOTHER	209
	Introduction	209
	Hypoglycaemia	210
	Other medical problems of the IDM	212
	Post-discharge care	214
	Reference	214
	Further reading	214
16	INFECTION	215
	Susceptibility to infection	215
	Cross infection	217
	Prolonged rupture of the membranes	221
	Minor infections in neonates which can be treated on the postnatal ward	222
	Severe neonatal infection	227
	Congenital infections	227
	Reference	231
17	JAUNDICE ON THE POSTNATAL WARD	232
	Bilirubin physiology	232
	Kernicterus	232
	Practical bilirubin chemistry	233
	Clinical implications of jaundice	234
	Rapid onset (Day 1) jaundice	234
	Infection	237
	Physiological jaundice	238
	Prolonged neonatal jaundice	239
	Investigation	241
	Treatment of neonatal jaundice	242
	Follow-up	246
	References	247

18	COMMON PROBLEMS IN THE WELL NEONATE	248
	Sequelae of birth	248
	Neurological problems	255
	Respiratory system	259
	Cardiac problems	260
	Mouth	262
	Gastrointestinal tract	263
	Genitourinary problems	269
	Lumps, bumps, tags and holes	272
	Pyrexial babies	275
	Pallor	276
	Plethora/polycythaemia	277
	Hypoglycaemia	277
	Hypocalcaemia	280
	Skin problems	280
	Limb abnormalities	285
	References	286

19	SERIOUS ILLNESS PRESENTING IN A PREVIOUSLY WELL NEONATE	287
	Respiratory problems	287
	Cardiovascular problems	290
	Neurological problems	292
	Serious infection	293
	Gastrointestinal problems	299
	Haemorrhage	301
	Sudden collapse	302

20	MALFORMATIONS	305
	Antenatally diagnosed structural malformations	305
	Postnatally diagnosed malformations	308
	Dysmorphic syndromes	309
	Down's syndrome	310
	Harelip, cleft palate, mid-line cleft palate	312
	Congenital dislocation of the hip	313
	Talipes	315

Metatarsus varus 317
Limb abnormalities 317
Ambiguous genitalia 318
Hypospadias 320
Dwarfs 320
Meningomyelocele 321
Care of lethal malformations 322
References 323
Further reading 323

21 DURATION OF STAY AND DISCHARGE 324

Normal babies 324
Small babies 324
Babies with malformations 324
Medical problems 325
Follow-up 326
Reference 328

INDEX 329

PREFACE TO SECOND EDITION

The majority of newborn babies, hopefully at least 90 per cent depending on local neonatal practice, are cared for in the postnatal wards and family bedrooms. These babies nevertheless require careful medical surveillance. They all have to be examined routinely, and this examination frequently reveals minor variations. These are usually normal or, if abnormal, the abnormalities are of no significance but nevertheless need to be recognised, correctly diagnosed and explained appropriately to the parents.

The babies also have to be fed, and no area of neonatal care results in more conflicting advice being given, or creates more maternal anxiety than this topic. Babies also may have minor medical problems such as sticky eyes or spots; they may be bruised, and a multitude of other minor problems may occur which need appropriate treatment.

Much to be recommended is the modern tendency to look after certain groups of babies, such as those who are slightly small-for-dates, born to diabetic mothers, or follow multiple pregnancies on the postnatal wards with their mothers.

The care of all these babies often falls within the remit of general practitioners, obstetric SHOs and, frequently, and most importantly, of midwives. In addition, many paediatricians-in-training have responsibilities for the care of babies on postnatal wards. This book is intended for all these groups.

Finally, throughout this book the neonate is referred to as 'he'. This sexism is to prevent tortuous isosexual phraseology and is also a tacit recognition that we males are the weaker sex and need more care and attention from the neonatal period onwards.

1995   **NRCR**

1

INTRODUCTION

—

'A human being is more likely to die on the first day of his life than on any other except the last one.'*

Although 50–60 per cent of pregnancies detected by maternal endocrine changes in the first 4–6 weeks fail, primarily early in the first trimester, the opening statement pithily emphasises that despite all the recent advances in perinatal medicine, and the fact that having a baby has never been safer for a mother or her baby(ies), in England and Wales, just under 1 per cent (8 per 1000 births) of all women who go into labour will produce either a stillborn baby or a neonate who dies in the first few days or weeks. About 2 per cent of pregnant women (20 per 1000 births or 1 in 50) will produce a baby with some malformation, and of those malformations 5–10 per cent (1–2 per 1000 births) will be rapidly fatal. Even more women – about 6 per cent (60 per 1000 or 1 in 16) – will produce a baby who needs to be admitted to a neonatal unit and who has an illness which may be fatal (and therefore is included in those enumerated above), but which in others will require the full range of modern neonatal intensive care with long-term artificial ventilation, detailed and meticulous haematological, biochemical, respiratory and cardiological monitoring and, in many cases, intravenous nutrition, before a usually neurologically intact survivor graduates from the neonatal intensive

---

*Aphorism of Professor J. A. Davis, Professor of Paediatrics in Cambridge 1979–1988.

care unit. Descriptions of the medical care of the 6–10 per cent of neonates who are ill are now the subject of an ever increasing selection of textbooks of neonatology (Taeusch *et al.*, 1991; Avery *et al.*, 1994; Fleming *et al.*, 1991; Roberton 1992, 1993): this book is concerned with the remaining 90–94 per cent.

THE NORMAL TERM BABY

The vast majority of neonates, about 85–90 per cent, are 'normal', healthy, full term babies who should never go anywhere near an intensive care unit (Chapter 10). Nevertheless, to say that such babies do not require expert nursing and neonatal care is seriously to misrepresent one of the most important areas of paediatric care, which should normally be given either on a postnatal ward (PNW), or in the parents' own home. The first section of this book, therefore, outlines the medical care of this patient, and the impact on him of maternal illness which has to be understood if appropriate care and unjustified mother–baby separation are to be avoided (Chapter 3).

Every neonate may need to be resuscitated. He must be fully examined at least once by a competent paediatrician, preferably in the presence of the mother who should be encouraged to air any anxieties she has about her baby, and these queries should only be answered from a position of knowledge. All neonates require routine aspects of care, such as prophylactic vitamin K (p. 77) and biochemical screening procedures (Chapter 8). All babies have to be fed, and there is probably no area of medical care where the patients' next of kin are left more confused by advice given to them by so-called experts.

Minor medical problems are common (20–30 per cent of all neonates become jaundiced). Other problems commonly encountered are sticky eyes, murmurs, a wide assortment of skin rashes and lumps and bumps, and multiple minor malformations such as birthmarks, undescended testes and accessory auricles or digits.

Confidence in managing all these aspects of neonatal care is required by everyone responsible for looking after newborn babies either in hospital or at home.

SPECIAL BABIES

A most important part of modern 'normal neonatal care' is the medical management of those babies (about 8–12 per cent of all live births) who are currently kept on the PNW, but who would, in the past, have been admitted to a neonatal unit (NNU). This includes the larger pre-term babies of 1.7–1.8 kg to 2.5–2.6 kg birthweight, small-for-dates (SFD) babies of similar birthweight, jaundiced babies and many with minor symptoms or feeding difficulties. In some hospitals all these neonates are lumped together on one PNW, often dignified with the grandiose and unjustifiable title 'transitional care'. I believe, however, that the majority of such babies can be perfectly adequately looked after with all the full term 3.5 kg specimens on a routine PNW. Nevertheless, such babies do need extra input from the nursing and medical staff. To say that they do not is a serious, potentially dangerous mistake. What is true, however, is that the extra effort which is required to look after these babies on a PNW is the best way to provide postnatal care for both the mother and her baby. The second part of this book describes that care.

REFERENCES

Avery, G.B., Fletcher M.A. and MacDonard M.G. (1994). *Neonatology*, 4th Ed. J.B. Lippincott, Philadelphia.

Fleming, P.J., Speidel, B.D., Marlow, N. and Dunn, P.M. (1991). *A Neonatal Vade-Mecum*. Edward Arnold, London.

Roberton, N.R.C. (Ed.) (1992). *Textbook of Neonatology*, 2nd Ed. Churchill Livingstone, Edinburgh and London.

Roberton, N.R.C. (1993). *A Manual of Neonatal Intensive Care*, 3rd Ed. Edward Arnold, London.

Taeusch, H.W., Ballard, R.A. and Avery, M.E. (1991). *Diseases of the Newborn*, 6th Ed. W.B. Saunders, Philadelphia, London.

2

DEFINITIONS AND STATISTICS

GESTATION

TERM

A baby born between 37 and 42 completed weeks of pregnancy (i.e. 259–294 days) dated from the first day of the mother's last menstrual period. If this date is uncertain, accurate gestational age assessment can be obtained by ultrasonic fetal measurements which are nowadays usually carried out late in the first trimester or early in the second. Assessing gestational age by ultrasonic measurements, first carried out after 24–28 weeks gestational age, is fraught with difficulty, and in particular it is doubtful whether adjusting the estimated duration of pregnancy by 7–10 days (i.e. much less than the duration of one menstrual cycle) is justified on the basis of third trimester ultrasonic fetal measurements.

PRE-TERM, PREMATURE

A baby born before 259 days' gestation, irrespective of birthweight.

POST-TERM, POSTMATURE

A baby born after 294 days' gestation.

IMMATURE

This has no medical definition; the word should be used for its non-specific meaning as defined in the Oxford English Dictionary: 'not mature, not perfect or complete, unripe'.

DYSMATURE

This term should not be used as it is confusing and has different meanings to different paediatricians. These range from a non-specific description of a scraggy baby to, in some instances, the bloated babies of diabetic mothers.

BIRTHWEIGHT

LOW BIRTHWEIGHT (LBW)

'Prematurity' was defined by the World Health Organisation (WHO) in 1950 as any baby weighing <2.50 kg at birth, irrespective of gestation. Although it is now recognised that many infants of this weight are SFD (see below) the weight criterion has become internationally accepted as the definition of LBW.

VERY LOW BIRTHWEIGHT (VLBW)

Never formally defined, but by convention the term is currently used to describe babies weighing <1.50 kg at birth.

EXTREMELY LOW BIRTHWEIGHT (ELBW)

Never officially defined, but by common assent is currently used to describe babies weighing <1.00 kg at birth.*

---

*Professor Ann Greenough of King's College Hospital, London, has coined the term ILBW (incredibly low birth weight) for babies < 0.75 kg. Whether this receives the accolade of everyday usage will have to await the test of time!

BIRTHWEIGHT FOR GESTATION

Centile charts for the birthweight of infants of both sexes and many races born in different geographical and social settings have been produced. For British babies several authors and sources have produced their own data of which Fig. 2.1 and Table 2.1 (Yudkin *et al.*, 1987) are representative and recommended.

In general, in paediatrics, the normal range of any measurement such as height, weight, head circumference or more recherché measurements such as the distance between the eyes or the size of the testes is taken to be either between the 3rd and 97th centiles or between plus and minus two standard deviations from the mean (average) measurement.

The 3rd centile means that 3 per cent of the normal population are smaller than the measurement, and 97 per cent are bigger; the converse is the case for the 97th centile. Standard deviation is mathematically derived from the average of measurements in a sample, and the range and number of measurements in the sample – the greater the range and the smaller the number, the bigger the standard deviation. Plus or minus two standard deviations corresponds to the 2.3rd and the 97.7th centile, so the values are very similar to the 3rd and 97th centiles.

When talking about birthweight for gestation, however, some neonatologists believe that different limits should be set, in particular using a cut-off for SFD at the 5th or even 10th centiles (p. 181). I do not believe that this is justified (Chapters 11 and 18) and the definitions below are based on that belief.

SMALL-FOR-DATES, LIGHT-FOR-DATES

A baby whose birthweight is on or below the 3rd centile for his gestation, the centile data being based on

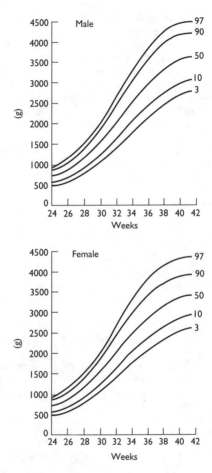

FIGURE 2.1 Birthweight centiles by gestational age (from Yudkin *et al.*, 1987).

TABLE 2.1 Birthweight smoothed means and centiles by gestational age

Gestational age (weeks)	Smoothed centiles (kg)				
	3rd	10th	50th	90th	97th
Males and females					
24	0.51	0.60	0.74	0.88	0.97
25	0.55	0.63	0.79	0.95	1.03
26	0.60	0.70	0.87	1.05	1.14
27	0.68	0.79	0.98	1.18	1.28
28	0.77	0.91	1.12	1.34	1.48
29	0.91	1.04	1.30	1.56	1.69
30	1.06	1.20	1.49	1.79	1.93
31	1.20	1.36	1.70	2.04	2.20
32	1.36	1.54	1.92	2.30	2.49
33	1.52	1.72	2.14	2.57	2.76
Males					
34	1.69	1.91	2.38	2.86	3.08
35	1.85	2.10	2.61	3.13	3.37
36	2.01	2.28	2.83	3.38	3.64
37	2.17	2.45	3.03	3.61	3.88
38	2.31	2.60	3.20	3.81	4.09
39	2.45	2.75	3.35	3.96	4.25
40	2.58	2.87	3.47	4.07	4.36
41	2.70	2.97	3.55	4.13	4.40
42	2.70	2.98	3.55	4.12	4.39
Females					
34	1.67	1.87	2.33	2.80	3.00
35	1.81	2.03	2.53	3.04	3.26
36	1.96	2.20	2.73	3.26	3.50
37	2.12	2.36	2.91	3.46	3.71
38	2.26	2.51	3.07	3.63	3.89
39	2.38	2.65	3.21	3.78	4.05
40	2.49	2.76	3.33	3.90	4.16
41	2.59	2.86	3.42	3.97	4.24
42	2.60	2.87	3.43	3.98	4.25

From Yudkin *et al.*, 1987

an appropriate population sample. It is inappropriate to plot babies from Nepal where the people are short, commonly malnourished and live at 15 000 ft, on charts from tall, over-fed, sea level Anglo-Saxons!

LARGE-FOR-DATES, HEAVY-FOR-DATES

A baby whose birthweight is on or above the 97th centile for his gestation, using weight charts from an appropriate population (see above).

EMBRYO

The developing human in utero from the formation of the inner cell mass in the blastocyst 1 week after fertilisation of the ovum, up until the 12th week of pregnancy calculated from the first day of the LMP. Given that ovulation occurs roughly half-way through the menstrual cycle, the embryo is in fact only 9 weeks old when a women is 12 weeks pregnant (i.e. 10 weeks from conception minus the initial week for the formation of the blastocyst).

FETUS

The developing human in utero from the end of the embryonic period until delivery.

POST-CONCEPTIONAL AGE

This term is sometimes used when describing preterm babies and refers to their age since birth plus their gestation. Thus a 6-week-old baby, born at 25 weeks gestation, has a post-conceptional age of 31 weeks. The term post-conceptual is sometimes used; this is not correct English.

VIABILITY

In some countries there is a statutory definition of viability. This is not the case in Britain. However, the Infant Life Preservation Act of 1929 recognised the state of 'capable of being born alive'. The change in the Abortion Act in 1990 and recent court judgments carry the implication that babies of 24 weeks are viable, as indeed are those less than this who are capable of being born alive.

LIVEBORN

Any baby who after delivery shows signs of life. This is again a very woolly area legally, since even very immature fetuses of 16–20 weeks will have a heart beat, move and make some respiratory effort if they are delivered appropriately, though immaturity of most organ systems, specifically the lungs, gastrointestinal tract, skin and reticulo-endothelial system precludes survival at such gestations. A sensible attitude is to limit the term 'viable' to babies beyond some preset gestation at which long-term intact survival can occur, say, 22 weeks (154 days) or 24 weeks (168 days). All such babies should have a birth certificate and, if they die, a death certificate.

STILLBORN

The law in Britain changed on 1 October 1992 to include as stillbirths all babies of 24 weeks gestation (168 days) or more who are dead when expelled from the birth canal. Such a baby receives a stillbirth certificate. Until this date only babies of 28 weeks or more were registered as stillbirths.

This definition of stillbirth creates two anomalies:

1 Stillborn babies (i.e. Apgar 0, see pp. 67–8) can in some cases be resuscitated: they then qualify for a birth certificate, and if appropriate a death certificate. They do not get a stillbirth certificate.
2 Although babies born alive below 24 weeks gestation are registered as live births, if they are born dead they are not registered as stillbirths, but are merely abortions either spontaneous or induced and do not receive any certification.

PERINATAL, NEONATAL, INFANT

PERINATAL PERIOD

The perinatal period (as far as birth and death registration and statistics are concerned) is now from 24 weeks of gestation (168 days) to 7 days of postnatal age, irrespective of birthweight and gestation at delivery. The term is, however, more loosely but quite justifiably applied clinically to the latter half of pregnancy plus the first week or so of life.

NEONATAL PERIOD

The first 28 days of life, irrespective of the gestation at delivery. The neonatal period is commonly divided in to the early neonatal period (0–7 days) which is included in the perinatal period for data collection (see below), and the late neonatal period (8–28 days) which is not. The period 29–365 days is often referred to as the post-neonatal period.

INFANT, INFANCY

A baby from the moment of birth to his first birthday (365 days), irrespective of his gestation at delivery.

MORTALITY STATISTICS

These are routinely collected in most parts of the world, but the level of accuracy varies from place to place. This is largely due to the obvious problems in the developing countries of ascertaining all live births, particularly in rural areas, never mind the problems of ascertaining those that are stillborn or die. In England and Wales the data is collected and analysed by the Office for Population, Censuses and Surveys (OPCS) from the birth certification done by the parents, and stillbirth and death certificates provided by the hospital, correlated with the statutory birth notifications completed on all births by the birth attendant (midwife or doctor).

In the developed world there are still problems in producing accurate and comparable mortality statistics and collecting satisfactory data on fetal wastage at gestations below 28 weeks, and at birthweights below 1.00 kg. The World Health Organisation recommends that data should be collected on all babies ≥ 22 weeks/gestation, and weighing ≥ 0.50 kg at birth. The change in stillbirth notification to 24 weeks from 1 October 1992 will improve accuracy, but problems remain with babies of 22–23 weeks and weighing less than 600 g.

The fallback position recommended by the WHO is to give 'standard perinatal statistics' and to report data only on births (live or still) weighing ≥ 1.00 kg or, if the birthweight is unavailable, at gestations of 28 weeks or more. This has much to recommend it, and in current labour ward and perinatal practice in Britain it is highly unlikely that any such live or still-birth would not be registered.

STILLBIRTH RATE

This is the number of stillbirths (i.e. 24 weeks gestation or above) irrespective of birthweight expressed per 1000 total births, i.e. stillbirths plus live births. The most recent (1993) figure for England and Wales is 5.3/1000 total births higher than in recent years because of the change in stillbirth definition.

NEONATAL MORTALITY RATE

This is the number of live born babies, irrespective of birthweight or gestation (so long as they get a birth and death certificate), who die in the first 28 days of life expressed per 1000 live births (LB). The most recently available rate in England and Wales is (1993) 4.1/1000 LB. The neonatal mortality rate (NNMR) is usually sub-divided in to the early NNMR from 0–7 days (currently 3.2 per 1000 LB in England and

Wales) and the late NNMR from 8–28 days (currently 0.9/1000 LB in England and Wales). The NNMR showed considerable improvement till the mid-1980s (Fig. 2.2) with a tendency to level off in the last 5–10 years.

PERINATAL MORTALITY RATE

This is the stillbirth rate plus the early (0–7 days) neonatal mortality rate expressed per 1000 in total births. The most recent data in England and Wales is 8.9/1000 total births, and like the NNMR has showed a gratifying fall till the mid-1980s (Fig. 2.2) but has risen with the recent change in still birth definition.

CORRECTED NEONATAL AND PERINATAL MORTALITY RATE

On the basis of the WHO recommendations, this is the NNMR and PNMR excluding all babies > 1.00 kg at birth. Such figures are not available nationally in

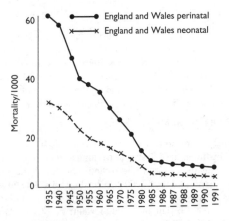

FIGURE 2.2 Neonatal and perinatal mortality in England and Wales 1935–85.

England and Wales, but the data for Cambridge is given in Table 2.2. This shows that the death of a live-born baby weighing > 1.00 kg at birth is now exceptional and in fact that most such deaths are due to malformations.

TABLE 2.2 Standard perinatal mortality, Cambridge Maternity Hospital, 1975–92 (i.e. only data in neonates and stillbirths > 1.00 kg birthweight)

	PNM	NNM	NNM†
1975	18.0	8.7	*
1980	10.7	6.5	*
1985	5.3	2.5	*
1986	5.0	3.5	*
1987	5.8	3.9	1.6
1988	4.2	2.2	1.8
1989	7.4	4.1	3.8
1990	3.7	2.3	0.3
1991	6.8	4.5	1.8
1992	3.1	2.2	1.1

*Data not available. †Excluding congenital malformations.

INFANT MORTALITY RATE

This is the number of babies who die in the first year of life (0–365 days) expressed per 1000 live births. It is currently (1993) 6.2/1000 live births, and comprises the NNMR (see above), plus the post-neonatal mortality rate (29–365 days) currently 2.1/1000 live births. The post-neonatal mortality rate, in particular that component due to cot death, has begun to drop significantly in the last 2–3 years.

REFERENCE

Yudkin, P.L., Aboualfa, M., Eyre, J., Redman, C.W.G. and Wilkinson, A.R. (1987). New birthweight and head circumference centiles for gestational ages 24–32 weeks. *Early Human Development* 15, 45–52.

3

THE EFFECT OF MATERNAL ILLNESS, BAD HABITS OR THERAPY ON THE BABY

MATERNAL ILLNESS

ABDOMINAL TRAUMA

Concern is always expressed that abdominal trauma from assault, falls and motor vehicle accidents, particularly with inappropriately placed seat belts, may cause uterine damage, placental abruption and thus fetal compromise or premature labour. However, though well-attested examples of adverse outcomes exist, they are the exception rather than the rule (Dahmus and Sibai, 1993). However, fetomaternal bleeding may occur occasionally causing serious fetal anaemia or hypovolaemia, but more important, rhesus sensitisation in rhesus negative women. Appropriate prophylaxis should therefore be given in such cases. In all cases the fetus should be monitored for 24–48 hours after the incident, and if all is well the mother may then be discharged.

ACUTE ILLNESS

Illness in the pregnant woman can have many effects on her fetus, though in general these are non-specific in one of four ways:

If these problems occur around the time of

RESULT	CAUSE
• Miscarriage, fetal death, spontaneous onset of pre-term labour	Acute febrile illness, e.g. flu, meningitis. Any severe and acute illness, e.g. acute appendicitis, trauma, haemorrhage, myocardial infarction.
• Severe fetal CNS damage	Similar to the above, but marginally less severe, so that uteroplacental blood flow is compromised sufficiently to cause fetal cerebral ischaemia, but not enough to cause fetal death. Also caused by specific neurotropic pathogens, e.g. rubella, CMV, toxoplasmosis, varicella, herpes.
• Intrauterine growth retardation (IUGR)	Almost any chronic maternal illness, e.g. urinary infection, malaria, malnutrition, chronic renal disease and most of the complications of pregnancy such as recurrent ante-partum haemorrhage (APH) and pre-eclamptic toxaemia (PET). Maternal bad habits – smoking, drinking, drug abuse.
• Need to effect early delivery (or termination) in the interests of maternal health.	Severe life threatening maternal disease, e.g. leukaemia, renal failure or severe complications of pregnancy such as eclampsia.

delivery, it is usually easy to decide after delivery whether or not it will be appropriate for the mother to breast-feed. If a prompt recovery is anticipated, then the baby can be transiently bottle-fed, or put on bank breast milk until the mother is well enough to feed him. However, if a prolonged maternal illness is likely, then it is sensible to start the baby on bottle-feeding (p. 140, Chapter 9). The gestation of the baby is of little relevance, since if he is born prematurely it is of considerable benefit to him if his mother maintains her lactation if at all possible, and provides her own expressed breast milk for him.

The problems with perinatal maternal infectious disease are discussed on p. 25.

ALLERGIC DISEASES

(see p. 132)

ASTHMA

For the vast majority of asthmatic women neither their illness nor its treatment has any deleterious effect on the pregnancy or their ability to breast-feed their baby. If there is a problem for asthmatic mothers, it is an unjustified unwillingness to use vigorous antiasthma therapy during pregnancy and lactation. Severe, steriod-dependent asthmatics, because of chronic lung disease, may produce slightly growth-retarded babies. None of the drugs used to treat asthma is a contraindication to breast-feeding.

AUTOIMMUNE DISORDERS

Any condition due to maternal or immune disease mediated by IgG antibodies may be transmitted to the fetus. This includes conditions like haemolytic anaemias and immunologically mediated skin disease such as herpes gestationis. Other common autoimmune disorders – myasthenia (p. 30), thrombocytopenia (p. 28), systemic lupus (p. 34), and thyrotoxicosis (p. 35) – are considered elsewhere in this chapter.

CARDIAC DISEASE

In the 1990s heart disease in pregnancy is commonly the woman with corrected congenital heart disease, coronary artery disease, prosthetic heart valves or even post-heart (and lung) transplantation, rather than the classical problems with rheumatic heart disease. The increased plasma volume of pregnancy may precipitate heart failure and limit exercise tolerance in all these groups but this can usually be controlled medically. Few fetal or neonatal complications of maternal heart disease are seen, though IUGR may be seen with severe maternal heart disease or corrected severe congenital heart disease (e.g. Mustard correction of transposition of the great vessels). However, pregnancy can usually be allowed to continue in all these situations with every prospect of a successful outcome except in women with either primary pulmonary hypertension or Eisenmenger's syndrome (pulmonary hypertension secondary to a large left to right shunt). Of such mothers 30–50 per cent die in the puerperium with, for reasons that are not entirely clear, a progressively falling blood pressure and PaO_2.

Most drugs required for the management of cardiac disease can be given safely in pregnancy with the exception of the anticoagulants of which Dindevan and warfarin are potentially teratotogenic and will also anticoagulate the fetus. They should, therefore, be substituted by heparin during the first 12–16 weeks and for 2–3 weeks before delivery.

Labour in women with heart disease is often short and easy, but should never be allowed to be prolonged; perinatal problems for the baby are rare, and breast-feeding is not contraindicated.

CHRONIC LUNG DISEASE – CHRONIC BRONCHITIS, BRONCHIECTASIS

If severe, this might cause some fetal growth retardation. Antibiotics, if required, should be chosen which do not have transplacental or neonatal effects (p. 43). Breast-feeding is not contraindicated.

CYSTIC FIBROSIS (CF)

Women with CF whose lung function is poor, should be discouraged from becoming pregnant since not only is their baby likely to become motherless early in life, but for the mother, the intra-abdominal mass of pregnancy compromises diaphragmatic action, reduces lung volume and accelerates the deterioration of her lung function. For those with milder disease who are meticulous with their physiotherapy and nutritional management, there should be few problems, and if antibiotic prophylaxis is being used, drugs which affect the fetus should be avoided (p. 43). Even if the mother produces large amounts of infected sputum containing organisms such as *Pseudomonas aeruginosa*, there is no risk from these to her baby unless he also has CF.

Since 1:20 of the general population are CF heterozygotes, the mother has a 1:20 chance of marrying a carrier, and therefore a 1:40 chance of having a baby with CF. Antenatal diagnosis should, therefore, be offered.

Although earlier studies suggested that the breast milk from mothers with CF had a dangerously high sodium content, this was due to a faulty collection technique. The salt content of breast milk in a mother with CF is normal, and other things being equal, there is no contraindication to her breast-feeding.

DIABETES

(see Chapter 15)

EPILEPSY

Pregnancy normally poses no problems for epileptic women, though it probably increases their susceptibility to convulsions. In part, this is because their plasma anticonvulsant levels fall due to the haemodilution and more rapid drug metabolism in pregnancy. Occasionally, a severe prolonged seizure may, by causing profound maternal hypoxia and decreased uteroplacental oxygen transfer, result in fetal neurological damage.

Infants of epileptic women do have an increased incidence of malformations. Although the issue is not entirely settled, this seems more likely to be due to the anticonvulsant drugs than the epilepsy itself. Trimethadione (Tridione) causes IUGR, mental deficiency and an odd flat face with mid-facial hypoplasia. Since this drug is no longer a mainline anticonvulsant, its use in pregnancy is unlikely. Sodium valproate and carbamazepine are associated with neural tube defects and dysmorphic features and should either be avoided in pregnancy, or appropriate fetal screening with α-fetoprotein or ultrasound carried out. Phenytoin in some cases causes IUGR, harelip and cleft palate, and digital anomalies, but mental defect is very rare. For most women on phenobarbitone the risk of fetal damage is remote. It is therefore both necessary (for the mother) and safe to continue these anticonvulsants in pregnancy.

Postnatally the baby may develop a form of 'abstinence' though this is usually mild and transient, with nothing more than a little jitteriness, some irritability and poor feeding which do not require treatment. Maternal treatment, with phenobarbitone and phenytoin in particular, may cause severe neonatal haemorrhagic disease, and appropriate vitamin K prophylaxis must be given after delivery (p. 77).

Finally, prenatal exposure to phenobarbitone activates fetal glucuronyl transferase so that neonatal jaundice is less likely in such infants. So effective is this, that it has been suggested as antenatal therapy in women likely to produce a jaundiced baby, though it is doubtful if it is ever clinically justified.

Postnatally there should be no major constraints on the epileptic mother and how she cares for her baby, though she should obviously be cautious about situations where, were she to have a fit, the baby might come to harm, for example, during the baby's bath, or when he is being carried downstairs.

Breast-feeding is not contraindicated. The amount

of anticonvulsant which gets through into the baby's bloodstream is usually so small that it has no effect; however, if the mother is on high doses, particularly of phenobarbitone, and her breast-fed baby is really dozy and not feeding adequately, bottle-feeding should be started.

There are no contraindications (contrary to popular belief) to full immunisation of her baby including the pertussis component.

GASTROINTESTINAL DISEASE

Acute severe intestinal diseases such as Crohn's or ulcerative colitis may cause fetal loss. These diseases in their severe chronic form, and some cases of coeliac disease, may produce premature delivery or mild growth retardation. However, the prognosis for pregnancy in women with these diseases is, in general, excellent.

Since the tendency to develop coeliac disease is inherited, and aggravated by the early introduction of gluten into the diet, all mothers, never mind those with coeliac disease, should be encouraged to delay the introduction of gluten (wheat) containing cereals in to the baby's diet until he is at least 3 months old, and, if given gluten earlier, not to bottle-feed since this may increase the likelihood that the bowel will absorb the food antigens whole (Auricchio *et al.*, 1983).

HAEMOGLOBINOPATHIES

Thalassaemia major or homozygous sickle cell disease, HbSC or HbSThal, makes getting pregnant and staying pregnant difficult, though with improved long-term management of these diseases more affected women are having full term pregnancies. Pregnancy in heterozygotes has few if any problems.

For parents who are known homo- or heterozygotes accurate antenatal diagnosis is now available, but if, despite these facilities, a homozygous baby is born he has few problems in the neonatal period, since in the presence of HbF ($\alpha_2\gamma_2$) he is not dependent on HbA ($\alpha_2\beta_2$), and both sickle cell anaemia and thalassaemia are β chain disorders. Alpha-thalassaemia is rarely a problem in Britain.

HYPERTENSION

This is probably the single most common medical complication of pregnancy either on its own or as pregnancy induced hypertension (pre-eclampsia). In the latter, multi-organ involvement occurs in the mother with damage among others to the liver and the CNS (eclamptic convulsions).

When severe, it may predicate pre-term delivery with all that that entails, and in less severe cases a small-for-dates baby will be born at or near term. Both may suffer transient postnatal hypotension as a result of maternal drug therapy. Thrombocytopenia is also reported in such babies, but rarely if ever poses a clinical problem.

IRON DEFICIENCY

Maternal iron deficiency seems to have remarkably little effect on the fetus, the neonate's haemoglobin or the breast milk iron content. Even in the presence of severe maternal iron deficiency, iron supplies to the fetus or to the breast are maintained, and mean that the baby is not at risk from iron deficiency (Murray *et al.*, 1978).

MALIGNANT DISEASE

About 1:500 women are likely to develop malignant disease while pregnant (Table 3.1, Jacob and Stringer, 1990). In some cases, initial surgical treatment and local radiotherapy can be instituted without compromising the pregnancy; in others, such as cervical carcinoma, therapy is incompatible with continuing

TABLE 3.1 Estimated incidence of cancer per 1000 pregnancies (from Jacob and Stringer, 1990)

Site	Incidence
Cervix	1.00
Breast	0.33
Melanoma	0.14
Ovary	0.10
Thyroid	?
Colorectal	0.02
Leukemia	0.01
Lymphoma	0.01

pregnancy. In general, the prognosis for malignant disease diagnosed during pregnancy is no worse for identical stages of the disease. However, in several conditions, characteristically carcinoma of the breast, since the disease is often more advanced at diagnosis during the pregnancy, the ultimate outcome may appear worse.

An increasing number of women are now becoming pregnant after successful treatment of malignant disease in childhood or adolescence, and males who have survived such disorders are fathering babies. As might be expected, fertility is reduced in those who received chemotherapy or radiotherapy that affects the gonads, and women who have received abdominal radiotherapy, particularly for Wilms' tumour, have smaller and more premature babies. However, otherwise the outlook is excellent.

In the neonatal period babies of both groups of parents should be checked if the parental malignancy has a genetic component, and breast-feeding is contraindicated if the mother is on cytotoxic drugs. Otherwise the neonatal course of such babies is normal.

MALNUTRITION

Severe maternal malnutrition will result in the birth

of SFD babies, but the growth restriction is relatively mild. Giving nutritional supplements to chronically malnourished women in the developing world also has a surprisingly small effect in increasing birthweight. There is evidence to suggest that periconceptional maternal malnutrition causes an increased incidence of fetal malformations.

In the postnatal period the maternal malnutrition has to be much more severe that anything likely to be seen in Britain before it compromises the mother's ability to breast-feed. However, to sustain lactation optimally a mother should eat an extra 300–500 kCal worth of food per day over her basic requirements, the bigger intake being necessary for women who put on little weight in pregnancy.

MATERNAL INFECTIOUS DISEASE

Those conditions which can cause congenital infections such as rubella, CMV, toxoplasmosis, syphilis and malaria are described on p. 227. This section will concentrate on the neonatal impact of maternal infectious disease present at the time of delivery or developing in the immediate neonatal period (Table 3.2). Serious maternal infections early in pregnancy, apart from those causing congenital infection,

TABLE 3.2 Effect of perinatal maternal infections and their effect on the ability to breast-feed

Illness	Access to normal baby and ability to breast-feed	Treatment to baby
Acute enteric infections (cholera, typhoid)	Nil during acute phase, mother too ill	Nil, encourage breast-feeding if possible; immunise infant if appropriate
*Acute respiratory infection (RSV, flu)	Access with masking and hand washing: breast-feeding allowed	Nil
Chlamydia	No restrictions	Nil if baby is asymptomatic, but see p. 224

TABLE 3.2 Contd

Illness	Access to normal baby and ability to breast-feed	Treatment to baby
CMV	No restrictions on access or breast-feeding	Nil
*Gastroenteritis	Access with meticulous hand washing	Nil
Hepatitis A	No restriction, but meticulous hand washing	250 mg of standard immunoglobulin to baby
Hepatitis B	No restriction. Breast-feeding not contraindicated if full immunisation given	200 i.u. of high titre hepatitis B immuno-globulin stat, immunise baby with HBV vaccine stat plus boosters at 1 and 6 months
Hepatitis C	No restriction	Nil officially recommended, but 250 mg standard immunoglobulin may minimise the risk of intrapartum transmission
Herpes simplex (genital)	No restriction, but meticulous hand washing and gloves	Acyclovir orally to mother (see also p.219)
*Herpes simplex (labial, whitlow, etc.)	No restriction, but mother to wear face mask and to treat her lesions with acyclovir	None, unless symptomatic, when herpes must be excluded
HIV (see p.230)		
Leprosy	No restrictions	Continue maternal treatment
Malaria	No restrictions on access or breast-feeding if mother's general health acceptable	Test infant's blood for parasites especially if mother has falciparum malaria or if the infant develops symptoms; treat congenital infection with chloroquine
*Measles	No restrictions	Give 250 mg normal immunoglobulin to infant (hyperimmune if available)
*Mumps	No restrictions	Nil

TABLE 3.2 Contd

Illness	Access to normal baby and ability to breast-feed	Treatment to baby
Rubella	No restrictions	No problem to neonate, but keep mother away from other antenatal patients
Sexually transmitted diseases (gonorrhoea, syphilis)	Access with meticulous hand washing; no restrictions on breast-feeding if mother being treated	Assess baby carefully to check that he is not infected, in which case treat, especially with maternal syphilis (Zenker and Berman, 1991) and give eye prophylaxis (p. 76)
*Skin infections (boils, impetigo)	Access: meticulous hand washing; antibiotics to mother	Nil
*Streptococcal illness or carriage	No restrictions (see p. 221). Meticulous hand washing and masking, especially for group A strep. respiratory infection	Nil
Toxoplasmosis	No restrictions	Treat the baby (p. 228)
Tropical diseases (trypanosomiasis, schistosomiasis, filariasis)	Usually no restrictions	Nil, but consult local tropical diseases hospital if infant symptomatic
*TB — open	No restriction if mother's general health satisfactory; drugs do not pass in sufficient quantity into breast milk to contraindicate breast-feeding (Snider and Powell, 1984)	INAH to infant; BCG at 6 months if infant PPD negative or give INAH resistant BCG at once
TB — closed	As above	As above; normal BCG routine to neonate
Ureaplasma colonisation	No restrictions	Nil
*Varicella	Access restricted until	Give 250 mg ZIG to

TABLE 3.2 Contd

Illness	Access to normal baby and ability to breast-feed	Treatment to baby
	lesions crusted; mother gowned, masked and gloved	infant if maternal disease < 7 days pre-delivery; consider acyclovir
Zoster	Access	Nil, baby immune from transplacental IgG

*Conditions where mother may have access to her own baby, but not allowed into the NNU or to have access to other babies.

may have the non-specific deleterious effects outlined on p. 17.

If a mother is acutely ill with an infectious disease around the time of delivery, she may be too ill to undertake breast-feeding, and there is always the risk that she could transmit the infection to her baby. In such situations, the baby should be bottle-fed until that risk is past. However, in general, acute infections are not a contraindication to breast-feeding (Table 3.2).

MATERNAL THROMBOCYTOPENIA

(Burrows and Kelton, 1993)

Maternal thrombocytopenia is usually either an incidental association with pregnancy or due to maternal autoimmune idiopathic thrombocytopenic purpura. In the first group, neonatal thrombocytopenia is never a problem, whereas in the second there is an antiplatelet IgG in the mother which can cross the placenta and cause fetal and neonatal thrombocytopenia. This may still happen if the mother is asymptomatic during pregnancy either because she is on steroids or has had a splenectomy in the past. Women who are asymptomatic, on no drugs, or had a splenectomy some years ago are particularly likely to slip through the net and not be identified until their baby develops petechiae.

In both situations vaginal delivery can be allowed, though difficult rotational forceps or Ventouse delivery should probably be avoided.

Once the baby is born, he should be managed expectantly, unless bleeding (as opposed to purpura/petechiae) is a problem. If it is, the baby should be transferred to the NNU where the options are steroid therapy, intravenous immunoglobulin, exchange transfusion or a platelet transfusion.

Transplacentally acquired IgG has a half life in the neonate of about three weeks, and as the level falls the neonatal platelet count gradually rises and is usually normal by 4–6 weeks of age, though spontaneous haemorrhage is very rare after 7–10 days.

There is, of course, no contraindication to breast-feeding, even if the mother is on steroids.

These babies *must* be differentiated from those where the mother has some systemic disease complicated by an immune thrombocytopenia (e.g. SLE v.i.), and from babies with alloimmune (isoimmune) thrombocytopenia in which the mother's platelet count is normal but the baby becomes thrombocytopenic due to platelet antigen incompatibility between him and his mother. In such cases, prenatal and intrapartum cerebral haemorrhage are major risks and may be preventable by maternal treatment with steroids or immunoglobulin. Postnatally, the baby also requires NNU admission and treatment with steroids, immunoglobulin or washed maternal platelets.

NEUROLOGICAL DISORDERS

(see also epilepsy)

Women with a multitude of chronic neurological disorders including multiple sclerosis, many myopathies, Wilson's disease, Huntington's chorea and paraplegia on the basis of trauma or neural tube defects may well become pregnant. Other than the genetic implications of those conditions which are inherited, and obstetric problems due to weakness, neonatal problems are unusual except in women with two muscle disorders, dystrophia myotonica and myasthenia.

Dystrophia myotonica

This condition is inherited as an autosomal dominant. The increasing severity in successive generations and, in particular, the severe manifestation seen in babies of relatively mildly affected women is now known to be due to expansion of a triplet repeat (cytosine-thymine-guanine) up to several thousand times as the abnormal gene on maternal chromosome 19 is transmitted to the ovum. About 50 per cent of such infants are stillborn, born prematurely or suffer severe neonatal respiratory problems aggravated by their muscular weakness. The outlook is poor both for neonatal survival and long-term CNS and IQ development. In some cases, the problems in the neonate may be the first indication of the disease present in a mild form in the mother.

Myasthenia gravis

This condition is due to antibody to the acetylcholine receptor on the motor end-plate. The antibody is in the IgG class and is transmitted transplacentally to the fetus who presents in the neonatal period with marked hypotonia and poor sucking. This condition occurs in 10–20 per cent of the infants of affected women and should, therefore, be anticipated; the diagnosis in the neonate can be confirmed by an improvement in neonatal movement and activity in response to 1 mg of intramuscular edrophonium (Tensilon test). The baby may need to be treated with pyridostigmine for 4–6 weeks until the transplacental IgG has disappeared.

PARATHYROID DISORDERS

In the rare pregnant woman with hyperparathyroidism and hypercalcaemia, the resulting marked fetal hypercalcaemia will suppress the fetal parathyroids, so that marked neonatal hypocalcaemia may occur in the first week of life. This may cause convulsions. If such a case is recognised, daily monitoring of the neonatal plasma calcium should be undertaken and supplementary calcium gluconate and vitamin D given.

PHENYLKETONURIA (PKU)

If women with PKU intend to become pregnant, they must be started on diet preconception or early in the first trimester as soon as the first period is missed, otherwise exposure of the embryo to high plasma phenylalanine levels will result in microcephaly, mental defect and congenital heart disease in the infant. There are no neonatal problems, irrespective of the mother's dietary history, unless congenital heart disease is present, but if she was hyperphenylalaninaemic during early pregnancy, she should be counselled about the poor prognosis for her infant.

The baby will be screened for PKU in the usual way (Chapter 8). There is no contraindication to breastfeeding, even though the breast milk has a high phenylalanine content, and the baby is an obligate heterozygote, often with moderately high phenylalanine levels. However, these normally settle without getting up to the levels seen in PKU, and no treatment is required.

PSYCHIATRIC DISORDERS

Women with mild psychiatric disorders rarely pose any problem during pregnancy or the puerperium, though stress and depression increase the incidence of low birthweight and prematurity (McAnarney and Stevens-Simon, 1990). In women with severe psychiatric disorders, doubt may be cast on their ability to care for their babies. Planning the appropriate care for the baby may require careful long-term assessment of the mother's capabilities in collaboration with her psychiatrist, GP, social services, and her partner. In rare cases, taking the baby into care may be the only safe recourse. For women with severe postnatal depression, supportive out-patient and if necessary in-patient care in a mother and baby psychiatric unit is usually successful.

Occasionally, the baby of a mother taking a large amount of pyschotropic drugs may have withdrawal syndrome in the early neonatal period. However, this is usually mild with transient jitteriness, irritability and poor feeding. No treatment is usually required.

Most of the drugs used in psychiatry are not a contraindication to breast-feeding, and if the mother wishes to breast-feed, this should be allowed. If, however, the baby becomes sedated or fails to thrive due to high levels of drugs in the breast milk, then bottle-feeding should be started. Maternal therapy with lithium is, however, contraindicated antenatally, since it is a teratogen causing congenital heart disease, and postnatally it enters the breast milk in large amounts and causes marked neonatal sedation.

PYREXIA OF UNKNOWN ORIGIN (PUO)

A mother with an intrapartum pyrexia should be assumed to have an infection until proved otherwise. Her baby at birth will always be pyrexial since the fetus in utero always has a temperature about 0.5–1°C higher than its mother. If the infant is asymptomatic at delivery, routine swabs and a blood culture from the neonate should be taken, and Gram stains done on a maternal high vaginal swab and a neonatal ear swab. So long as the baby can be adequately supervised on a PNW with his mother, he should not be given antibiotics. Should he have any symptoms, however, these should be attributed to infection till proved otherwise; he should be admitted at once to the neonatal unit, fully worked up for infection and started on large doses of broad spectrum antibiotics.

If there is a possibility that the infection is viral, as opposed to bacterial, consideration should be given to infusing the baby with intravenous immunoglobulin. In symptomatic neonates whose condition rapidly deteriorates in the 4–6 hours postnatally, treatment with immunoglobulin and an exchange transfusion with fresh adult blood are indicated (p. 293).

RENAL DISEASE

Most forms of renal disease, including renal infection, nephrotic syndrome, chronic nephritis and the presence of a renal transplant, can cause obstetric problems, with hypertension and IUGR. Of chronically haemodialysed or transplanted women who get pregnant, no more than 50 per cent will have a normal term delivery. The effect of maternal antihypertensive therapy is discussed on p. 47.

Once the baby is born, however, apart from problems of prematurity or of the SFD baby, and transient hypotension (p. 23), no specific problems arise, though if the mother has an inherited form of renal disease, including chronic pyelonephritis secondary to reflux nephropathy, appropriate investigation of the neonate is indicated, usually by ultrasound scan of the kidneys.

Breast-feeding is not contraindicated unless the mother is taking immuno-suppressive drugs following a renal transplant.

RHEUMATIC DISORDERS

Other than potential problems from the drugs used (p. 48), women with these disorders and their newborn babies cause no particular neonatal problems. Indeed women with rheumatoid arthritis often feel better when pregnant.

SPHEROCYTOSIS

(see also p. 237)

This is an autosomal dominant condition, so an affected parent has a 50 per cent chance of transmitting it to his or her offspring. If a parent (particularly the father) had a splenectomy in childhood and is now fit and asymptomatic, his family history is frequently missed. Neonates with spherocytosis usually present within the first 24–48 hours with marked jaundice, which is Coombs' test negative and which will often need phototherapy and occasionally an exchange transfusion. The diagnosis should always be considered in an uninfected baby with a marked jaundice Coombs' test negative presenting in the first few days of life (p. 237).

Examination of the blood film in the neonatal period is less useful than in older patients with spherocytosis, since some spherocytes are present in other neonatal haematological problems, and neonates with spherocytosis do not have many spherocytes in their peripheral blood film. However, once the diagnosis is confirmed, often on the basis of the positive family history, the baby should be started on maintenance folic acid, 1 mg daily.

STOMAS

In women with stomas, be they ileostomies, colostomies or ureterostomies, there is in general no contraindication to pregnancy or breast-feeding either on the basis of the stoma or the underlying disease for which the procedure was carried out.

SYSTEMIC LUPUS ERYTHEMATOSUS

(Lancet, 1991)

For patients with active disease, fertility is reduced, and if they conceive major problems may develop. In patients with inactive disease the condition may relapse during pregnancy, and a further group of patients may present for the first time while pregnant. Treatment, including the use of steroids and cytotoxics, must be continued through pregnancy, and is not associated with fetal side-effects such as malformations. Active disease, with involvement of the renal and placental vasculature often with hypertension, will cause fetal problems, including fetal death, prematurity and IUGR. In addition, if the mother carries the anti-Ro antibody it crosses the placenta, attaches to the myocardial conducting tissues and may cause congenital heart block. This is usually detected antenatally because of a fixed fetal bradycardia in the 40–80 beats/min range but occasionally this will not be noticed until the woman is in labour, or even postpartum. If the heart rate is very slow, the baby may be in heart failure and may eventually need pacing.

As well as these cardiac problems, the neonate may have thrombocytopenia, a haemolytic anaemia and transient neonatal rashes all due to transplacental passage of antibodies from the mother. If any of these are a problem, they can usually be promptly controlled by steroids, exchange transfusion or appropriate replacement transfusion. However, this is rarely indicated, and the baby usually makes normal neonatal progress.

Breast-feeding is not contraindicated.

THYROID DISEASE

Thyrotoxicosis

The thyroid stimulating immunoglobulins (TSIG) present in exophthalmic Graves' disease, like all IgG, can cross the placenta. In the fetus they will stimulate the thyroid, causing fetal and neonatal thyrotoxicosis. This problem can occur in a woman cured of thyrotoxicosis in the past, but who still has elevated levels of TSIG. For the thyrotoxic pregnant female, drug therapy (but not radioiodine) should be used, giving the smallest dose which controls her symptoms: surgery is rarely indicated. Managing her disease this way should cause neither fetal hypothyroidism nor goitre, and indeed the transplacental drug may usefully control the fetal hyperthyroidism.

Fetal thyrotoxicosis causes tachycardia, commonly IUGR, and even intrauterine death. Neonatally the infant can develop all the features of thyrotoxicosis but this only occurs in about 1:100 infants of thyrotoxic mothers, and these are probably the 1 per cent with the highest titre of the thyroid stimulating immunoglobulins. Infants of thyrotoxic mothers should not be admitted routinely to an NNU, but should be carefully watched on PNW for early signs of thyrotoxicosis, including tachycardia, irritability, poor feeding, weight loss, exophthalmos, a goitre and heart failure. These symptoms can be present at birth or develop during the first 7–10 days. They are more likely to be delayed if the mother was receiving antithyroid medication which had partially controlled the fetal thyrotoxicosis. The neonate can become very ill very quickly and if symptoms do develop he should be admitted at once to the neonatal ward for treatment, usually using all three of Lugol's iodine, propanolol and propylthiouracil and also treating heart failure, if present.

Breast-feeding for the thyrotoxic mother treated by drugs is not contraindicated as long as she is on treatment with propylthiouracil, iodine or propanolol, since these do not cross in to the EBM in sufficient quantity to cause neonatal thyroid suppression. If any anxiety exists, however, neonatal thyroid function can always be tested. She should not breast-feed if she has recently received radioiodine treatment.

Thyrotoxic babies need careful follow-up; a few remain thyrotoxic, some develop craniosynostosis and several have developmental delay.

Hypothyroidism

Mothers who are hypothyroid in pregnancy may produce babies who are pre-term, but there are no other problems.

TOXOPLASMOSIS

If a mother seroconverts in the first 15–20 weeks of pregnancy, serious malformation is a possibility and termination should be considered. After 20 weeks' gestation, serious fetal CNS damage is rare but the mother should be treated with spiramycin alternating with sulphadiazine plus pyrimethamine (Remington and Desmonts, 1990) (p. 229).

VITAMIN DEFICIENCIES

The only one of importance is vitamin D. Women with a poor dietary intake, often combined with minimal exposure to sunshine because of climate, clothing or racial pigmentation, may be vitamin D deficient in pregnancy. In Britain women from the Indian sub-continent are particularly at risk.

As a result of the maternal hypovitaminosis D, the neonate may be small-for-dates, have decreased skull ossification and may develop hypocalcaemia in the first week with jitteriness or convulsions which usually respond to calcium supplements. It is worthwhile, therefore, supplementing all at-risk women with 400 units of vitamin D daily during pregnancy, since this will prevent neonatal morbidity.

The breast milk in unsupplemented, at-risk women is also very low in vitamin D, and since their babies are likely to have received very little vitamin D transplacentally, if a mother intends to breast-feed, her baby should receive Abidec 0.6 ml (400[u] vitamin D) daily, until an adequate mixed diet is established. Regular exposure of the baby to sunlight for no more than 30 minutes per day will also prevent rickets.

MATERNAL SUBSTANCE ABUSE

ALCOHOL

Alcohol is a teratogen and there is now clear evidence that women consuming throughout pregnancy two standard drinks per day are more likely to produce babies with features of the fetal alcohol syndrome; the more that is drunk and an indulgence in binge drinking, the more severe the fetal abnormality. While the counsel of perfection may be for women to avoid alcohol throughout pregnancy, acceptable evidence does not exist to proscribe the occasional social consumption of a couple of glasses of wine with dinner!

Postnatally, the group of women likely to produce babies with fetal alcohol syndrome should probably be encouraged to bottle-feed. In other breast-feeding women, there is no evidence to suggest that a glass of sherry has anything other than a mutually calming and soothing effect on both her and her baby, though it may transiently reduce milk intake (p. 43).

DRUG ADDICTION

It is important not to limit evaluation of the infant of a drug addict just to the effects of the drug. Most such mothers have major socio-economic problems and they are a group specifically at risk from all sexually transmitted diseases including hepatitis B and HIV. Malnutrition and alcohol abuse may also be a problem. They often produce low birthweight, ill babies requiring admission to the neonatal unit, but if the baby is well after birth and mature enough, he should be on the postnatal ward with his mother. If the abstinence syndrome is mild, he can be managed on the postnatal ward, but if severe with intractable vomiting or seizures, the baby should be admitted to the neonatal unit.

Opiates

The main neonatal problem following maternal opiate addiction is the abstinence syndrome, the symptoms of which are neatly summarised in Fig. 3.1. Withdrawal syndrome is not inevitable, and its severity and duration are related to the dose and type of opiate taken. Large-dose heroin addiction is likely to result in major problems within the first few days, whereas with low-dose methadone programmes no symptoms may occur, or they may be mild and last for weeks or even months.

It is important to remember not to give naloxone during labour ward resuscitation of asphyxiated neonates born to opiate addicted mothers; this may precipitate an acute abstinence syndrome.

Treatment of abstinence requires good nursing care, swaddling, a quiet environment and small frequent feeds. More severe symptoms can be controlled with methadone or non-narcotic drugs like chlorpromazine.

Cocaine

Maternal abuse of cocaine causes major problems to the fetus, with an increased risk of prematurity,

Wakefulness
Irritability
Tremulousness, temperature variability, tachypnoea
Hyperactivity, high-pitched cry, hyperacusis, hypertonus
Diarrhoea, disorganised suck
Respiratory distress, rhinorrhoea, rub marks
Apnoeic attacks
Weight loss or failure to gain weight
Alkalosis – respiratory
Lacrimation

FIGURE 3.1 Neonatal problems following maternal opiate addiction.

intrauterine growth retardation and vascular accidents damaging the brain, gut, renal tract and limbs; abruptio placentae is more common. However, if the baby is born alive without these problems, he does not seem to suffer abstinence syndrome, but recent long-term follow-up studies show some developmental delay.

Cannabis

There is now an extensive literature on maternal use of this drug which shows that it has little if any deleterious effect on the fetus.

TABLE 3.3 Non-narcotic drugs which may cause withdrawal syndrome

Alcohol	Magnesium sulphate
Barbiturates	Meprobamate
Benzodiazepines	Pentazocine
Bromide	Phencyclidine
Diphenhydramine	Phenothiazines
Glutethimide	Theophylline
Lithium	Tricyclic antidepressants
Local anaesthetics	

From Rylance, 1992.

Other drugs

A wide variety of drugs affecting the CNS are abused by women in pregnancy (Table 3.3). In general, these drugs have few neonatal effects other than to cause a mild abstinence syndrome which, if indicated, can be managed as outlined above for opiates.

Breast-feeding

The decision about whether breast-feeding is allowed is a complex one. If the mother is HIV positive or continues off a treatment programme, breast-feeding is contraindicated in developed countries. In other situations, it can be continued, but if feasible the concentration of drug in the breast milk should be measured.

MATERNAL SMOKING

It is surely clear to everyone that smoking is unwise. Mothers who smoke more than 10–15 cigarettes a day will produce babies at term weighing 200 g less than controls, and with a 50 per cent higher perinatal mortality.

Postnatally, the breast-fed baby of a smoker has higher levels of the various toxic products of cigarette smoking such as nicotine and cotinine in its blood (derived from breast milk) than does the bottle-fed baby of a smoking mother.

Smoking by the mother is also statistically correlated with a higher incidence of cot death, asthma and lower respiratory tract infection in her baby in the first year of life. Most interestingly, recent studies show lung function abnormalities within the first few weeks in infants of smoking mothers, suggesting that lung damage occurs prenatally.

MATERNAL DRUG THERAPY

In general, although there are many theoretical anxieties about the teratological effect of drugs and their deleterious pharmacological effects on the fetus in utero, in practice, considering that pregnant women take on average 10–12 drugs during pregnancy, surprisingly little harm has been reported to result from this, apart from the spectacular Thalidomide tragedy. The few drugs with well-established teratogenic effects are listed in Table 3.4, and these drugs should obviously be avoided during pregnancy. The problems of many drugs are considered above under the heading of the disease for which they are used, but some more generally used drugs also have implications for the neonate.

It can be assumed that all drugs that get into the mother's bloodstream, whether administered orally or by the parenteral route, will get into her

TABLE 3.4   Recognised teratogens

Drug	Defects
Antineoplastic drugs	Odd appearance, ↓DQ, IUGR
Androgens, progestogens	Masculinisation of the female fetus
Warfarin	Conradi type syndrome
Anticonvulsants	
Phenytoin	Odd appearance, hypoplastic nails, ↓OFC, facial clefts
Tridione	Odd faecies, ↓OFC, ↓IQ
Valproate, Carbamazepine	Neural tube defects, dysmorphism
Lithium	Congenital heart disease (Ebstein's)
Tetracycline	Enamel hypoplasia
	Tooth and bone staining
Metronidazole	Theoretical risk of mutagenicity at high dose
Thalidomide	Limb reduction defects
Antithyroid drugs	Goitre
Vitamin A analogues (e.g. Etretinate)	Severe multisystem congenital malformations

milk, and more is likely to get into her milk if the drug

1 is poorly protein bound in maternal plasma
2 has a small volume of distribution (i.e. stays in the plasma)
3 has a long plasma half life
4 is weakly ionised – and therefore not ionised in plasma
5 is lipid soluble
6 is of low molecular weight (e.g. not a hormone like insulin)

The concentration of drugs in milk is usually less than 10 per cent of the maternal plasma levels and often in the 1–2 per cent range. The amount ingested by the neonate will therefore be small, and the effect of this on the baby will be further reduced by deficiencies in absorption and first-pass metabolism in the neonatal liver.

For most drugs, therefore, it is safe for the baby to breast-feed. However, if the mother is taking large doses, the baby may be affected, showing sleepiness or sedation with a wide variety of drugs acting on the CNS, or jitteriness and irritability with anti-asthma drugs such as methylxanthines or β-mimetics.

ALCOHOL

Alcohol readily gets into breast milk and recent evidence suggests that following the mother having an alcoholic drink the baby takes less milk at the next feed – the cause of this is uncertain, but the milk undoubtedly smells and tastes different.

ANTIBIOTICS

Administration of sulphamethoxazole to the neonate increases the risk of kernicterus by displacing bilirubin from its albumin binding site. On this basis, it is recommended that long-acting sulphonamides are not given to a pregnant woman in the immediate pre-delivery period, nor to lactating mothers. There is, however, no evidence that transplacental or breast milk sulphonamides have ever caused kernicterus in a neonate.

Tetracyclines administered to the mother in the second and third trimester are incorporated into fetal dental enamel and bone, discolouring them and, in the case of the teeth, causing enamel hypoplasia; they should not, therefore, be used. They have, in any case, few therapeutic uses in the pregnant woman.

Streptomycin can cross the placenta and cause fetal deafness but other drugs are now available for treating TB, though rifampicin may be teratogenic and should be avoided in the first trimester. There is no evidence that giving the other ototoxic aminoglycosides to a pregnant woman has ever caused deafness in the baby.

Since metronidazole is a mutagen in high doses breast-feeding should be discontinued for 12–24 hours after single high dosage to mother.

ANTICONVULSANTS

(pp. 20–1)

ANTICOAGULANTS

Warfarin is a teratogen (Table 3.4) and both it and phenindione cross the placenta and anticoagulate the fetus by inhibiting the synthesis of vitamin K dependent factors. These drugs should be stopped 4 weeks before delivery, and if the mother still needs anticoagulation she should be swapped to subcutaneous heparin, which does not cross the placenta. If the mother delivers before the anticoagulants are stopped, vitamin K must be given intravenously at birth and the baby's coagulation status checked afterwards to ensure that it has been corrected. Phenindione gets in to the breast milk in sufficient quantities to anticoagulate the neonate, and is therefore contraindicated in lactating women. Warfarin, however, does not get in to breast milk, and is therefore the anticoagulant of choice in the puerperium.

ANTITHYROID DRUGS

(p. 36)

ASPIRIN

Aspirin is a prostaglandin synthetase inhibitor and so theoretically may prolong pregnancy and cross the placenta with fetal cardiovascular effects. It has also been used in extensive low-dose trials to prevent preeclampsia. When used in low dosage, it does not compromise neonatal coagulation. For the occasional women taking large therapeutic doses of aspirin neonatal prophylaxis with vitamin K is essential.

CAFFEINE/METHYLXANTHINES

Caffeine (as social beverages) and methylxanthines get into the fetus and into breast milk. There may be a rise in the fetal heart rate, and neonatally the breast-fed baby of a coffee-drinking mother may be irritable or sleep poorly. Trial and error is the best way for the lactating mother to assess this potential problem.

CHLORMETHIAZOLE (HEMINEVRIN)

This potent anticonvulsant is used to control fulminating maternal pre-clampsia or eclampsia. It crosses the placenta easily and causes hypotonia and sedation in the neonate. In pre-term infants, in particular, this may be so marked that IPPV is required. There is no antidote, and the infant should be allowed to sleep it off.

Since the drug is only used in conditions which are potentially life threatening to the mother, her health is the imperative, and the paediatrician must be prepared to cope with the side-effects in the neonate.

CHLOROTHIAZIDE (AND HYDROCHLOROTHIAZIDE)

Antenatal maternal therapy may cause fetal thrombocytopenia and this differential should be considered in any neonate who presents with petechiae. There are, however, no problems with the use of these drugs in the puerperium, other than perhaps a reduction in milk formation.

CYTOTOXIC DRUGS

Theoretically these are contraindicated in pregnancy and lactation. However, there is an increasing number of women who have had organ transplants who have delivered normal babies having been immuno-suppressed throughout pregnancy with drugs like azathioprine and cyclosporin, and for such women it is difficult to envisage further damage should they breast-feed. However, therapeutic use of cytotoxic drugs is clearly incompatible with either continued pregnancy or lactation.

DIURETICS

These can get across into the baby and theoretically could cause dehydration, though this has never been reported. However, they may also reduce milk production, and their use should therefore be carefully controlled in lactating women.

EPIDURAL ANAESTHETIC

Detailed neurologiocal and behavioural assessment of newborn babies suggests that those delivered under epidural anaesthetic have marginally reduced responsiveness in the early neonatal period. This has been attributed to transplacental passage of the small amount of the epidural anaesthetic which is absorbed into the maternal bloodstream. Such effects are transient and have no clinical importance.

ERGOTAMINE

Theoretically this can cause vasospasm in the baby and vomiting, diarrhoea and convulsions have been reported in the babies taking this preparation via breast-feeding.

GENERAL ANAESTHETIC

Both the inhalational and intravenous anaesthetic agents may cause respiratory depression in the newly born neonate, and this may be aggravated by fetal hypocapnia secondary to maternal hypocapnia from mechanical over-ventilation of the unconscious woman. These effects on the neonate are aggravated if there is co-existing asphyxia. However, with modern intrapartum care and high-standard obstetric anaesthesia such problems are rare.

GLUCOSE

Excessive i.v. dextrose given to a woman during labour, for example as a vehicle for a tocolytic or an

oxytocic, may make her and her fetus hypergly-
caemic, resulting in rebound hypoglycaemia in the
neonate in the first few hours of life. If infants of
mothers who have had a free-flowing dextrose infusion in the latter part of labour develop any unusual
symptoms or signs in the first 4–6 hours of life, hypoglycaemia must be excluded.

HYPOGLYCAEMIC AGENTS

The oral hypoglycaemic drugs such as chlor-
propamide, tolbutamide and glibenclamide cross the
placenta and markedly stimulate the fetal islets of
Langerhans. As a result, prolonged and refractory
neonatal hypoglycaemia occurs after birth. These
drugs should not be given to pregnant women.
Although the literature is sparse, they should also be
avoided in lactating women.

HYPOTENSIVE DRUGS

Transplacental passage occurs with the antihyperten-
sion drugs commonly used in pregnancy. With
methyldopa and hydralazine, there seem to be few
maternal or fetal problems. The β-blocking drugs
such as propanolol and atenolol, and the combined
α- and β-blockers such as labetolol, have been widely
used in treating hypertension in pregnancy. In general they seem to be safe so long as everything is
going well (deSwiet, 1985). However, if the fetus
becomes asphyxiated, these drugs, in particular
labetolol, in theory compromise the fetal response to
asphyxia, and if they are being used, fetal monitoring in labour must be more than usually meticulous.

Captopril may cause fetal death in experimental animals and adverse fetal and neonatal effects have been
reported following its use in human pregnancy. It
should, therefore, probably be avoided in pregnancy.

The baby born to a mother taking antihypertensive
drugs has a transiently lower blood pressure than

controls, but this effect is short-lived and of little clinical significance in the larger infant over 34 weeks gestation and 2 kg birthweight. In sick VLBW infants born to women treated with these drugs for severe hypertension or pre-eclampsia, the additional hypotensive effects of the drugs in neonates in whom early neonatal hypotension is a bad prognostic sign should be promptly recognised and treated with volume expansion or dopamine.

Most of these drugs, however, can be used safely in lactating women since so little is passed to the neonate in the breast milk that it is of no consequence. However, atenolol, sotalol and acebutolol are present in breast milk in higher concentrations and should probably be avoided.

LAXATIVES

With the possible exception of phenolphthalein derivatives, laxatives do not get into breast milk and have no effect on breast-fed infants.

NARCOTIC ANALGESICS

The popularity of these drugs for intrapartum analgesia is falling with the increasing use of epidurals. However, in association with intrapartum asphyxia, drugs like pethidine can cause marked respiratory depression at birth. Establishing adequate ventilation is always the priority in this situation, followed by naloxone (p. 66). Narcotics are very slowly cleared from the neonatal circulation and may be present for 5 days. To avoid prolonged sedation and poor feeding in such babies a large dose of naloxone (0.1 mg/kg) should be given after the resuscitation is completed, and the infant is breathing satisfactorily.

NON-STEROIDAL ANTI-INFLAMMATORY DRUGS

(see also tocolytics)

These drugs, which are prostaglandin synthetase

inhibitors, cross into the fetus, and if their use is prolonged may close the fetal ductus and cause neonatal persistent pulmonary hypertension. When used i.v. as tocolytics they also cause fetal/neonatal renal failure. If their use is essential in a pregnant woman with severe arthritis, the lowest acceptable dose must be used. There is no contraindication to their use during breast-feeding.

ORAL CONTRACEPTIVES

These will not harm the baby but oestrogen containing products are likely to reduce breast milk production by about 100 ml per day.

OXYTOCICS

The effects on the neonate of intravenous oxytocin or prostaglandin E used to induce labour remain controversial. Babies born after induction of labour are undoubtedly more likely to be jaundiced than those produced by spontaneous labour. Whether this is due to the oxytocin, some aspect of the labour which it induces, or just to relative immaturity, i.e. the induced fetus is not yet ready for delivery, has not been elucidated.

PSYCHOTROPICS/SEDATIVES

These drugs all cross the placenta and may cause the neonate to be sleepy, feed poorly and even become hypothermic, the latter being particularly a problem with diazepam. These effects may last 48–72 hours because the drugs are cleared slowly from the neonatal circulation. Since there are no specific antidotes, the only option is to avoid the use of these drugs in pregnant women if at all possible, and in particular, they should not be used for sedation during labour.

Breast-feeding is possible for most mothers on most psychotropic and sedative drugs. However, if the baby does become sleepy, breast-feeding should be stopped. The exception is lithium which, being a small molecule, gets into milk and the baby in high concentrations. Mothers taking lithium should not breast-feed.

RADIOPHARMACEUTICALS

Radioactive agents used therapeutically (e.g. I^{131}) or diagnostically (e.g. Ga^{67}) should not be given to pregnant or lactating women.

STEROIDS

Not only do these drugs do little harm to the baby, they may actually mature many of his body systems, in particular his surfactant synthesis. Postnatally women on low dosage oral steroids or inhaled steroids may breast-feed.

TOCOLYTICS

Various drugs have been used to inhibit uterine contraction, and all have been associated with fetal and neonatal effects. In addition, the over-exuberant intravenous administration of such drugs to the mother is often inadvertently associated with maternal and fetal fluid overload, hypoglycaemia (pp. 277–9) and hyponatraemia. Since these drugs are only going to be used in pre-term labour they are, to some extent, outside the scope of this book since they are unlikely to affect infants cared for on the postnatal ward. However an outline of their effects will be given.

Alcohol

This is rarely used as a uterine relaxant in the UK; in the USA excessive alcohol administration for this purpose occasionally resulted in neonatal sedation with a high plasma alcohol, as well as neonatal hypoglycaemia and lactic acidosis.

β-adrenergic agents

Many have been used, but currently ritodrine and terbutaline are the most popular. They may cause fetal tachycardia, hypokalaemia and a lower glomerular filtration rate and, because they raise maternal glucose, may cause reactive neonatal hypoglycaemia. Clinically significant problems, however, seem to be rare.

Magnesium sulphate

This is widely used in the USA, but rarely in the UK. It may cause neonatal hypotonia and intestinal sedation ileus.

Prostaglandin synthetase inhibitors

The jury is still out on whether these drugs, which are good tocolytics but close the fetal ductus and cause fetal and neonatal renal failure, should be used. They have not caught on in the UK.

REFERENCES

Auricchio, S., Follow, D., deRitis, G., Giunta, A., Marzorati, D., Prampolini, L. et al. (1983). Does breast-feeding protect against the development of clinical symptoms of coeliac disease in children? *Journal of Pediatric Gastroenterology and Nutrition* **2**, 428–433.

Anonymous (1991). Systemic lupus erythematosis in pregnancy: Editorial. *Lancet* **338**, 87–88.

Burrows, R.F. and Kelton, J.G. (1993). Fetal thrombocytopenia and its relation to maternal thrombocytopenia. *New England Journal of Medicine* **329**, 1463–1466.

Dahmus, M.A. and Sibai, B.M. (1993). Blunt abdominal trauma: are there any predictive factors for abruptio placentae or maternal-fetal distress? *American Journal of Obstetrics and Gynecology* **169**, 1054–1059.

deSwiet, M. (1985) Antihypertensive drugs in pregnancy. *British Medical Journal* **291**, 365–366.

Jacob, J.H. and Stringer, C.A. (1990). Diagnosis and management of cancer during pregnancy. *Seminars in Perinatology* **14**, 79–87.

McAnarney, E.R. and Stevens-Simon, C. (1990). Maternal psychologicial stress/depression and low birth weight.

American Journal of Diseases of Children **144**, 789–792.

Murray, M.J., Murray, A.B., Murray, N.J. and Murray, M.B. (1978). The effect of iron status of Nigerian mothers on that of their infants at birth and 6 months, and on the concentration of iron in breast milk. *British Journal of Nutrition* **39**, 627–630.

Remington, J.S. and Desmonts, G. (1990). Toxoplasmosis. In: Remington, J.S. and Klein, J.O. *Infectious Diseases of the Fetus and Newborn Infant,* 3rd Ed., Eds W.B. Saunders, Philadelphia, pp. 143–263.

Snider, D.E. and Powell, K.E. (1984). Should women taking antituberculous drugs breast-feed? *Archives of Internal Medicine* **144**, 589–590.

Zenker, P.M. and Berman, S.M. (1991). Congenital syphilis. Trends and recommendations for evaluation and management. *Pediatric Infectious Disease Journal* **10**, 516–522.

FURTHER READING

Rylance, G.W. (1992). Pharmacology. In: *Textbook of Neonatology,* 2nd Ed., Ed. Roberton, N.R.C. Churchill Livingstone, Edinburgh, London, pp. 1193–1212.

4

RESUSCITATION OF THE NEWBORN

—

With modern obstetric care, only a small percentage of newborn infants are not pink, vigorous and howling lustily by 1–2 minutes of age. About 5 per cent of all deliveries are apnoeic at 1 minute of age, and about a quarter of these will need intubation in the delivery room.

About 70 per cent of the infants requiring resuscitation are born following some complication of pregnancy or labour. A neonatal paediatrician should, therefore, always be present at such deliveries (Table 4.1).

TABLE 4.1 Deliveries which should be attended by a paediatrician

- Gestations < 36 weeks
- Instrumental or surgical deliveries (excluding Wrigley's forceps deliveries)
- Malpresentations
- Twins and higher multiples
- Fetal distress and meconium staining
- Rhesus incompatibility
- Antenatal ultrasonic evidence of malformation
- Obstetrician distress

CAUSES OF DELAYED ONSET OF REGULAR RESPIRATION

A frequent misconception is that delayed onset of respiration is the result of intrapartum asphyxia. However, many factors other than asphyxia can delay the onset of respiration after delivery (Table 4.2); several of these may be present in an individual baby. It is crucial to recognise, however, that if failure to establish respiration is *not* the result of asphyxia, adequate resuscitation must nevertheless be carried out at once, or all the biochemical and clinical consequences of asphyxia will immediately develop.

TABLE 4.2 Factors other than asphyxia which may delay the onset of respiration after delivery

- Drugs — depressing the CNS
- Trauma — especially to the CNS
- Prematurity — in particular surfactant deficient, stiff lungs
- Muscle weakness — due to prematurity or primary muscle disease
- Anaemia
- Congenital malformations — obstructing the airway or preventing lung expansion
- Sepsis, characteristically Group B streptococci (p. 293)
- Previous neurological damage in utero

PHYSIOLOGY OF ASPHYXIA

To understand the effects of asphyxia on both the fetus and the neonate, and in particular its role in delaying the onset of spontaneous respiration, it is convenient to consider chronic partial asphyxia and acute asphyxia separately.

CHRONIC PARTIAL ASPHYXIA

By far and away the more common clinical problem is the previously normal baby who suffers recurrent episodes of partial asphyxia during labour due to, for example, oxytocin induced hypertonic and incoordinate uterine contraction, or recurrent episodes of umbilical cord occlusion due to entanglement round a fetal part. During such episodes the fetus increases his blood pressure, becomes bradycardic, and the cardiac output is concentrated on the placenta, brain and myocardium. The fetal PaO_2 falls, and energy is produced by anaerobic metabolism of glycogen and glucose to lactate. Since the $PaCO_2$ also rises, a combined metabolic and respiratory acidaemia develops. These episodes may be transient and/or infrequent in which case the fetus makes a complete 'clinical' and biochemical recovery before the next one or before delivery. If such a baby is delivered immediately, his respiration may be depressed, and he will probably respond promptly to resuscitation and have few if any sequelae.

If these episodes persist or are prolonged, the fetus no longer recovers between each one, and gradually becomes hypotensive and profoundly acidaemic. Damage to many organ systems, including the brain, will occur – and despite prompt resuscitation after delivery, severe neonatal illness and/or permanent neurological sequelae will result.

ACUTE ASPHYXIA

In clinical practice this is relatively rare, but study of it in animals has been very useful in understanding the pathophysiology of asphyxia and our management of it. In newborn monkeys delivered in good condition by caesarean section, and then asphyxiated before the onset of breathing by sealing their heads in a bag of saline, after a few shallow 'breaths' without achieving any gas exchange the animals stop 'breathing'. This period of 'primary' apnoea may last 10 minutes. However, after 1–2 minutes in primary apnoea most animals start to gasp with increasing frequency and vigour, and then decreasing frequency and vigour until they literally reach the last gasp. Gasping lasts for 5–10 minutes after which the animal is again apnoeic (Fig. 4.1).

The heart rate falls rapidly after birth, rises slightly in primary apnoea and early in the phase of gasping, but then slows. Cardiac activity continues for 10 minutes or more after the last gasp. The period between

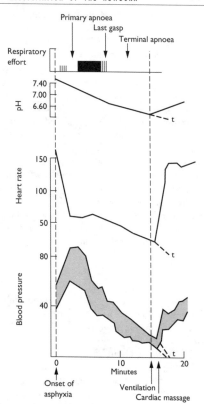

FIGURE 4.1 Adapted from Dawes et al. (1963).

the last gasp and cardiac arrest is known as secondary or terminal apnoea. A severe mixed acidaemia develops; by the end of terminal apnoea the $PaCO_2$ exceeds 13.5 kPa (100 mmHg), the H^+ exceeds 300 nmol/l (pH < 6.5) and the PaO_2 is unrecordable. Hyperkalaemia of more than 15 mmol/l develops.

The neonatal primate can therefore survive 20 minutes of complete oxygen deprivation. This is due to the large stores of glycogen in brain, liver and myocardium which can produce energy by anaerobic glycolysis, and also to the ability of neonatal brain to metabolise lactate and ketones (Settergren *et al.*, 1976).

The response to removing the bag of saline from the animal's head during the above experiment depends on the state of asphyxia. In primary apnoea, the apnoea will persist until the pH falls to that which provokes gasping, when the animal will inhale air or oxygen, and soon develop regular respiration. If the animal is gasping when the bag is removed, air or oxygen enters its lungs and a regular respiratory pattern develops. If the bag is removed in terminal apnoea, respiration will never occur. To resuscitate such an animal, positive pressure ventilation must be used. If the heart rate is very low (or has stopped), external cardiac massage will be necessary.

RELEVANCE OF ANIMAL EXPERIMENTS TO CLINICAL NEONATAL CARE

There is no reason to suppose that the human neonate would respond to asphyxia differently from animals. His response after delivery will depend on his pH. If his H^+ concentration is less than 55 nmol/litre (pH > 7.25), he will behave as though in the period of primary apnoea or gasping, and regular respiration will soon start. If his H^+ concentration has risen to 80–100 nmol/litre (pH 7–7.10), he may still breathe adequately, but particularly if there is some other complication such as heavy sedation or prematurity, the primary apnoea may be prolonged, or the gasping efforts may be too weak to establish alveolar ventilation. Still more severe intrapartum asphyxia will result in the delivery of an infant with an H^+ concentration above 100 nmol/litre (pH < 7.0) who is limp, bradycardic and in terminal apnoea.

The experiments on animal asphyxia have provided several other important pieces of data which help us to understand the behaviour and treatment of the human infant who is asphyxiated or apnoeic after delivery.

These include:

- The onset of gasping and therefore regular respiration can be expedited in primary apnoea by peripheral stimuli including rubbing the baby with a warm towel or sucking out his upper airway.
- Drugs adminstered to the mother including all commonly used sedatives and analgesics pass to the fetus and may prolong primary apnoea to such an extent that the acidaemia becomes severe, and the phase of gasping may never occur.

ASSESSMENT OF THE SEVERITY OF ASPHYXIA

THE APGAR SCORE

The traditional way of assessing the newborn is to use the Apgar score. This was devised by Dr Virginia Apgar (1953) and grades five clinical features with scores from 0 to 2 at one minute of age (Table 4.3). Although the one minute score has limitations as an index of asphyxia, it is undoubtedly an efficient measure of the need for resuscitation. There may be many causes for an infant having a low Apgar score at 1–2 minutes (Table 4.2), but whatever the cause, he requires active resuscitation as soon as possible. However, because of the limitations of the Apgar score, one should not just say that the baby had an Apgar of 5 at one minute, but should accurately describe the infant's condition. For instance, 'at one minute the infant was apnoeic, had blue hands and feet, a heart rate of 90 and normal tone; he grimaced when sucked out' or 'at one minute the infant was pink with a heart rate of 120 and gasped twice but

TABLE 4.3 Apgar score

Clinical feature	Score		
	0	1	2
Heart rate	0	< 100	> 100
Respiration	Absent	Gasping or irregular	Regular or crying lustily
Muscle tone	Limp	Diminished, or normal with no movements	Normal with active movements
Response to pharyngeal catheter	Nil	Grimace	Cough
Colour of trunk	White	Blue	Pink

he was limp and made no response to suction'. Both these situations score an Apgar of 5, but have entirely different clinical and physiological implications. The response to resuscitation should then be continued as a narrative in the baby's notes ending only when he is pink, breathing normally and active.

ASSESSING THE APNOEIC BABY

If a baby does not start to breathe, the crucial question is whether or not he is in primary or terminal apnoea. Infants in primary apnoea are usually in reasonable clinical condition with a heart rate near 100, good peripheral perfusion and body tone, although cyanosed and apnoeic (Apgar 5–7). Infants in terminal apnoea are more likely to be pale and apnoeic with little or no body tone or reflex response, and their heart rate is usually less than 60 (i.e. Apgar 1–3).

However, in many babies this diffentiation is not clear-cut, and if apnoea lasts for more than 2–3 minutes after delivery, active resuscitation is always indicated.

CORD BLOOD GAS ANALYSIS

The most satisfactory and accurate way of assessing whether or not a baby is asphyxiated at the moment of birth is measuring the blood gases and pH in a sample drawn from the umbilical artery in a section of the umbilical cord clamped off immediately after delivery. The results can be available within 5–10 minutes, and can then be extremely useful in planning further treatment.

RESUSCITATION

Unlike elsewhere in this book where I have been concentrating on what might be called the 'well-baby-care' aspects of neonatal medicine, the management of resuscitation of the newborn infant is described in considerable detail, and is very similar to the instructions given in *A Manual of Neonatal Intensive Care* (Roberton, 1993). This is because I believe that it is essential that everyone who takes responsibility for delivering a woman, even though she is at term and carrying an entirely normal pregnancy, must be able to resuscitate the baby who is unexpectedly severely depressed and apnoeic immediately after delivery.

Although all subsequent neonatal illnesses can be dealt with by transfer to a regional neonatal centre, it is irresponsible for any doctor or midwife to officiate during labour without being capable of carrying out the forms of resuscitation described in this chapter, or having someone with the necessary skills available within the same building.

PREPARATION

Do not be proud; if a very sick infant, or several infants, are expected or appear, call for help. In addition, ensure that you have adequate equipment and that it is working.

Equipment

- An adequate shelf on which to lie the infant.
- A supply of up to 5 litres/minute of oxygen for the face mask, bag and mask or endotracheal tube. Whichever method of administering oxygen is used the gas *must* be passed through a blow-off valve set at 30 cmH$_2$O.
- Adequate suction with a soft end on the sucker. The suction should not exceed 200 mmHg and, for routine use, should be set at 100 mmHg ($\equiv$ 136 cmH$_2$O) to prevent damage to the oropharyngeal mucosa. FG3–4 suction tubes are needed to clear the ETT, and FG8–10 tubes to clear the airway. Do not use mouth-held mucus extractors because of the risk of infection, especially HIV.
- An overhead radiant heat source, and sides to the resuscitation shelf to minimise the convective and radiant heat losses.
- A large stop-clock with a sweep second hand, since time passes very quickly in any emergency procedure.
- A mask for blowing oxygen over the face of the cyanosed but breathing baby.
- A bag and mask system for artificial ventilation, in general the Ambu and infant Laerdal systems are preferable (Field *et al.*, 1986). The easiest to use are masks with a pneumatic rim to obtain a tight face seal, connected to a sponge-filled, rapidly inflating bag. The mask must be detachable from the bag unit, and replaceable with a connector for an endotracheal tube. The bag and mask systems *must* be used in accordance with the manufacturer's instructions, otherwise dangerously high inflation pressures can be applied.
- A selection of baby-size oropharyngeal airways (sizes 00 and 000).
- At least two laryngoscopes (since one may fail at the crucial moment); which blade to have on the laryngoscope is a matter of individual preference, but generally speaking a straight-bladed one of the Wisconsin, Magill or Oxford Infant type is best.
- A selection of endotracheal tubes (2.5, 3.0 and 3.5 mm), either oral or nasal, though oral ones with a shoulder are easier to insert.
- Magill forceps for nasoendotracheal tubes.
- Appropriate devices for connecting the ETT to the resuscitation bag.
- A selection of syringes, needles and specimen bottles.
- Adhesive tape and a large pair of scissors.
- A stethoscope.
- Equipment for emergency cannulation of the umbilical vessels should also be on the trolley together with a thoracentesis set.

Drugs

The only drugs required on the trolley are:

Sodium bicarbonate (4.2%, 7.5% or 8.4%)	10 ml ampoules
THAM 7%	10 ml ampoules
Normal saline	10 ml ampoules
10% Dextrose	10 ml ampoules
Naloxone 0.4 mg/ml	2 ml ampoules
Vitamin K	1 ml ampoules

A small box should be included containing the following drugs which are occasionally needed in emergencies: frusemide, calcium gluconate, 1:1000 or 1/10 000 adrenaline, atropine.

Checklist

When preparing for a resuscitation always run through the following checklist:

- Read the mother's notes or get a history from the obstetrician about her medical/obstetric past, including the reasons for any surgical delivery, and also what drugs she has received during labour.
- Resuscitaire oxygen turned on and working. Blow-off valve presssure set at 30 cm H_2O.
- Clock wound up and working.
- Suction working at pressure of 100 mmHg; suction catheter attached.
- All the above equipment present, interchangeable and working.
- Go round and close all the doors and windows and turn off fans near the resuscitation trolley. The labour ward staff will hate you, but it is important to do this to prevent the infant becoming profoundly hypothermic, particularly if he is premature.
- Are there some warmed dry towels to wrap the baby in during resuscitation?

INITIAL ASSESSMENT OF THE INFANT

Start the clock the moment the baby is free from the mother's body (not when the cord is clamped). Assess the heart rate, respiration, colour and tone as soon as possible. For heart rate listen with a stethoscope – do *not* feel the cord since all you feel is your own heart beat pounding away in your finger tips. The baby will fall into one of four groups:

- fit and healthy, bawling lustily
- not breathing too well, but no immediate need for panic (5–6 per cent)
- obvious terminal apnoea – pale, limp and apnoeic, heart rate < 60 (0.2–0.5 per cent)
- dead but resuscitatable (< 0.1 per cent)

Fit and healthy

Leave this baby alone! Do not suck him out, since this traumatises the pharynx, and is a powerful vagal stimulus provoking a reflex bradycardia. Vigorous suction is based on the frequently held misconception that what is coming out of the baby's mouth is inhaled liquor. It is not; it is pulmonary fluid which has been in the lungs prior to birth, and it will do no harm if it stays there a few moments longer. If the upper airway is full of meconium, blood, antiseptic cream or some other extraneous material, the infant should be laryngoscoped and his mouth, larynx and trachea aspirated under direct vision.

The infant should be dried and wrapped in a warm blanket to minimise heat loss, given a dose of vitamin K, and given to his mother who should be encouraged to put him to the breast (see Chapter 9).

Snatching him away for some arcane medical ritual at this point is cruel and unnecessary – even the vitamin K can wait. In the first hour, babies are awake and alert, and this period is very important in establishing a close attachment between mother and baby. There is absolutely no need to bathe the infant at this time; it does him no harm to be covered in vernix or have some blood in his hair. Having a bath in a labour ward is a very efficient way of dropping even a healthy baby's body temperature to below 35°C.

Not breathing too well, but no immediate panic

For preterm infants (< 32–34 weeks' gestation) at risk from RDS there is no point procrastinating in this situation. Intubate them at once and get them pink and breathing as soon as possible. Such infants should probably stay intubated and on IMV until they are on the NNU and base line blood gases and X-rays have been done.

Most term infants will respond promptly to bag and mask resuscitation. Some, because they are slightly premature, drug depressed and/or respond poorly to bag and mask resuscitation may need to be intubated within the first 5 minutes. However, such babies usually respond promptly to just 2–3 minutes' IPPV, indicating that they are in primary apnoea and they can then be extubated. So long as they are active, breathing easily and pink by 10 minutes, they can go to the postnatal ward with their mother. For babies in poorer condition at birth or those who do not respond to simple bag and mask resuscitation follow Fig. 4.2.

Note the following:

- Bag and mask ventilation is difficult to do effectively, particularly in the infant who has never breathed and cleared his lungs of liquid, and this technique should therefore only be used in those babies who have made some, albeit inadequate, respiratory effort. To do bag and mask ventilation effectively, there must be a tight seal between the mask and the infant's face. Slightly extend his neck, and hold his jaw forward – an oropharyngeal airway may help.
- There is much to be said for using a simple Y connector attached to the endotracheal tube. It is safe, easy to use and has the advantage that a

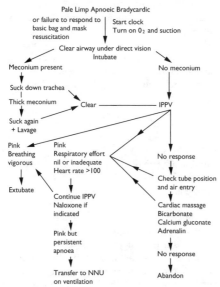

Pale Limp Apnoeic Bradycardic

or failure to respond to | Start clock
basic bag and mask | Turn on O_2 and suction
resuscitation

Clear airway under direct vision
Intubate

Meconium present — No meconium

Suck down trachea

Thick meconium → Clear → IPPV

Suck again
+ Lavage

Pink | Pink | No response
Breathing | Respiratory effort
vigorous | nil or inadequate | Check tube position
| Heart rate >100 | and air entry

Extubate | Continue IPPV | Cardiac massage
| Naloxone if | Bicarbonate
| indicated | Calcium gluconate
| | Adrenalin

| Pink but | No response
| persistent
| apnoea | Abandon

| Transfer to NNU
| on ventilation

FIGURE 4.2 Resuscitation of the newborn (from Gandy and Roberton, 1987, with permission).

long inspiratory time (>1 s) can be used, which is important in establishing a functional residual capacity.

- When resuscitating a baby by any method, make sure that the chest is moving and the lungs are being inflated. If this is not happening, you are doing something wrong, and if you are giving bag and mask ventilation it is safest to progress to intubation.
- To intubate a baby lie him flat or slightly extend his neck. Even moderate extension pushes the larynx into a very anterior position that makes it difficult to visualise. Insert the blade of the laryngoscope into the vallecula and pull the epiglottis forward to reveal the larynx. Press lightly on the

cricoid cartilage (with the fifth finger of the hand holding the laryngoscope), and the view of the larynx is improved.

- Mouth-to-mouth (plus nose) resuscitation is satisfactory in an emergency, but put in an oral airway and remember to extend the infant's neck. Blow very gently – just enough to ensure that the chest is being inflated.

- Only give naloxone after you have established respiration by what ever means necessary. *Never* give it to an apnoeic infant. Naloxone is best given intravenously. A dose of 0.1 mg/kg is given. Since pushing 1.0 ml of naloxone blind into the umbilical vein will probably not reach the systemic circulation, and giving a 'chaser' of normal saline is unsafe (p. 67), you either need to insert a venous catheter, find a peripheral vein or use the intramuscular route and wait several minutes for an effect.

- There is a tendency to give babies who respond slowly to resuscitation a few millimoles of bicarbonate and a few millilitres of albumin. This is bad practice: only give 'blind' bicarbonate to babies in terminal apnoea (v.i.). Otherwise only give i.v. base after blood gases have been measured and if the base deficit is > 10 mmol/l. It is doubtful if albumin is ever justified.

Apparent terminal apnoea

About 0.2–0.5 per cent of all deliveries are in this condition, and they represent about 5–10 per cent of all infants apnoeic at 2 minutes of age. Such a baby is severely asphyxiated. He will never breathe on his own unless you start him off. The longer you delay, the more profound the biochemical and physiological abnormalities, and the greater the likelihood of brain damage. Expeditious action is essential: follow Fig. 4.2, starting with intubation and IPPV.

Note the following:

- Avoid injecting drugs directly into the umbilical vein and if possible insert a venous catheter. Direct injection may:
  1 Swill an umbilical vein clot into the systemic circulation.
  2 Not reach the systemic circulation especially when giving small volumes (e.g. naloxone).
  3 Traumatise the umbilical artery causing haemorrhage and/or make subsequent arterial cathetisation difficult.
  4 Go directly into the umbilical artery causing spasm and ischaemia in the distribution of the iliac vessels.
- Most infants respond briskly to IPPV by going pink. However, if they are pink but not breathing by 3–5 minutes it can be assumed that they are severely asphyxiated and acidaemic.
- Babies with marked bradycardia (< 30–40) will benefit from a short period of ECM, and/or a dose of intratracheal adrenaline (v.i.).
- There is excellent data to show that brain damage in acidaemic infants who remain apnoeic despite adequate ventilation is related to the duration and severity of the acidaemia particularly in the CSF. Such infants should, therefore, be given i.v. base. Give 5–10 mmol of sodium bicarbonate i.v. over 2 minutes to all acidaemic infants who are still apnoeic after 5 minutes of IPPV.
- Most babies born in terminal apnoea will need to be admitted to the NNU and fully evaluated by blood gas, PCV, blood glucose and a CXR.

Dead

If the obstetrician is certain that the fetal heart was heard up to 10 minutes pre-delivery, it is always worth attempting to resuscitate the baby.

When confronted with a fresh stillbirth:

- Yell for help – since all cardiac arrest situations need more than one pair of expert hands.
- Give six to eight beats of external cardiac massage (ECM). This must be given properly. Prodding the sternum with two fingers is useless. The baby must be seized around the thorax with both hands; with the fingers of both hands supporting the thoracic spine, the sternum is powerfully depressed with both thumbs placed just below the sternal angle.
- Laryngoscope and aspirate under direct vision; intubate and give IPPV.
- Intratracheal adrenaline (0.5–1.0 ml of 1:1000) given at this point is rapidly absorbed into the pulmonary circulation, and thus reaches the heart.
- Continue ECM and IPPV; four beats of ECM to one lung inflation.
- Give 10 mmol of sodium bicarbonate intravenously – blindly if necessary.
- Try and get an ECG monitor and attach the leads.
- Insert a UVC.
- Assess: the infant will now be 3–4 minutes old. If no signs of life, give a further 10 mmol of sodium bicarbonate, 10 ml of 10 per cent dextrose, 0.5 ml of 1:1000 adrenaline and 1 ml calcium gluconate i.v. in that order. If these fail, repeat the sodium bicarbonate and give intracardiac adrenaline. If there is still no response, the infant will be 8–10 minutes old, so abandon resuscitation since neurologically intact survival has not been recorded in babies still asystolic aged 10 minutes.
- Once a heart beat is detected, the following drugs may be useful: naloxone (200 µg i.v.) (if relevant); atropine (0.1 mg i.v.) for persisting bradycardia; lignocaine (1–2 mg/kg i.v.) for ventricular tachycardia or fibrillation; calcium (1–2 ml of 10 per cent calcium gluconate) slowly under ECG control for hyperkalaemia and poor cardiac output. Glucagon (0.5 mg i.v. as a bolus), and dopamine

(5–20 µg/kg/minute i.v. by continuous infusion) are occasionally useful in an infant with a poor cardiac output.

- Admit to NNU continuing IPPV until base line blood gases, PCV, glucose, electrolytes and chest X-ray have been taken.

THE MECONIUM-STAINED INFANT

Meconium *staining* does not matter. *Inhalation* of meconium does. *A* paediatrician does not need to attend all deliveries where there is meconium-stained liquor unless there are other criteria such as fetal distress or instrumental delivery (Table 4.1.). Even if vigorous at birth such an infant should be laryngoscoped, meconium-stained liquor aspirated from his mouth and pharynx, and the trachea inspected to see if has inhaled any meconium. If he has, the trachea should be sucked out through the cords.

PROBLEMS WITH RESUSCITATION

THE INFANT WHO GOES PINK BUT DOES NOT START TO BREATHE

If by 20 minutes of age a neonate has made no spontaneous respiratory effort despite adequate oxygenation and empirical treatment with bicarbonate and naloxone, then further therapy should, if possible, be delayed until he is transferred to an NNU and blood gas analysis, blood glucose measurements and a chest X-ray been carried out. Remember that such babies may be suffering from some primary neurological disorder such as a cervical cord injury or a myopathy.

THE INFANT WITH NO RESPONSE TO IPPV

A few infants despite apparently adequate resuscitation will remain blue and bradycardic, with absent or grossly inadequate respiratory effort. In some cases, the reason will be obvious (e.g. lethal malformations). However, in infants who externally look normal the reason for the poor response is often some technical error in resuscitation. Therefore, check the following:

- If a bag and mask system is being used is there a poor seal around the face, and is the infant's chest moving?
- If intubated is the endotracheal tube in the trachea and not in the oesophagus?
- Is the endotracheal tube too small (a common mistake)? A 3.0 or 3.5 mm tube should always be used. Smaller tubes have a big internal resistance, allow a big airleak, and very easily get pushed in too far so that they lodge in a main stem bronchus, which is not only bad for overall ventilation, but carries the risk of rupturing the lobe and causing a pneumothorax.
- Is an adequate inflation pressure being applied? The blow-off valve may have become inadvertently reset at a low pressure.
- Is oxygen being given? Has the supply been disconnected or the reservoir removed from the bag and mask system?

If technical errors can be excluded:

- Is the asphyxia more severe than the initial clinical assessment suggested? Give a few beats of external cardiac massage, 0.5 ml of intratracheal 1:1000 adrenaline, and 5–10 mmol of intravenous sodium bicarbonate and continue IPPV. If possible, transfer to NNU for further evaluation.
- Is the infant premature and developing severe RDS or could he have congenital pneumonia? Increase the inflating pressure to 35 cmH$_2$O if possible and increase the ventilation rate. This virtually always improves the infant enough to allow transfer to the NNU.
- Is the infant very pale? Consider fetal haemorrhage into the mother, or from a placental separation, or from an injury to the placenta or a cord vessel dur-

ing delivery. Such infants may have lost more than half their blood volume. If the history is suggestive and the pallor seems due to anaemia, give 15–20 ml/kg of fresh uncross-matched O negative blood at once over 10 minutes. This will usually improve the baby enough for him to be transferred to a NNU where a more accurate assessment of the pallor can be made.

• Pneumothorax (see below).

THE VIGOROUS BUT CYANOSED BABY

A few infants are comparatively vigorous and active with a normal heart rate, often marked respiratory distress, yet remain very cyanosed. This situation strongly suggests some underlying structural problem in an (initially) unasphyxiated baby.

• Is there a diaphragmatic hernia, suggested by mediastinal shift, poor air entry on the left side (the usual side of the hernia) and a scaphoid abdomen? Get the infant into an NNU, on to a ventilator and X-ray him.

• Is there a pneumothorax? There is rarely time to confirm the diagnosis radiologically, but a fibre-optic light source may help. If the infant is deteriorating quickly, insert a wide bore needle into the second intercostal space in the mid-clavicular line. If a pneumothorax is present, the infant's condition will improve, and the needle can then be replaced by the insertion of a chest drain.

• Various lung malformations including the pulmonary hypoplasia of Potter's syndrome.

• Airway, lung or cardiac malformations which make the infant difficult to resuscitate are rarely surgically correctable, and are, therefore, usually fatal.

THE HYDROPIC NEWBORN

Always try to resuscitate hydropic neonates. Some recover, and all require careful evaluation to established a diagnosis which may be of critical importance to the mother's health (e.g. congenital infection) or be of importance for counselling for future pregnancies.

PARENTAL INVOLVEMENT

If, after active resuscitation by IPPV, the baby needs to be admitted to the NNU, show him to the parents and, if feasible, allow them to hold his hand or even cuddle him. Give the parents a brief résumé of what is happening, and aim to get them to the NNU as soon as possible to see their baby after his condition has stabilised.

REFERENCES

Apgar, V. (1953). Proposal for a new method of evaluation of newborn infants. *Anesthesia and Analgesia* **32**, 260–267.

Dawes, G.S., Jacobson, H.N., Mott, J.C., Shelley, H.J. and Stafford, A. (1963). Treatment of asphyxia in newborn lambs and monkeys. *Journal of Physiology* **169**, 167–184.

Field, D., Milner, A. and Hopkin, I.E. (1986). Efficacy of manual resuscitation at birth. *Archives of Disease in Childhood* **61**, 300–302.

Gandy, G.M. and Roberton, N.R.C. (1987). *Lecture Notes in Neonatology.* Blackwell Scientific Publications, London, pp. 113–126.

Roberton, N.R.C. (1993). *A Manual of Neonatal Intensive Care*, 3rd Ed. Edward Arnold, London, p. 369.

Settergren, G., Linblad, B.S., Persson, B. (1976). Cerebral blood flow and exchange of oxygen glucose, ketone bodies, lactate, pyruvate and aminoacids in infants. *Acta Paediatrica Scandinavica* **65**: 343–353.

FURTHER READING

Roberton, N.R.C. (1992). Resuscitation in the newborn. In: *Textbook of Neonatology.* Ed. Roberton, N.R.C. Churchill Livingstone, London and Edinburgh, pp. 239–256.

5

CARE OF THE NORMAL BABY IN THE DELIVERY SUITE

—

TEMPERATURE CONTROL

(Rutter, 1992)

Babies lose heat in four ways:

- conduction – to solid objects with which they are in contact
- convection – cooling due to air currents around the baby
- evaporation – taking out the latent heat of evaporation of water on the baby's skin
- radiation – to the nearest solid objects not in contact with the baby

A naked, liquor covered, newborn baby immediately after delivery loses heat by all methods. However, unless he is laid on a cold surface, *conductive* heat losses are small.

Convective losses

The air in the labour ward should be still and no cooler than 20°C; there should be no open doors or windows; fans or powerful air-conditioning vents should be well away from the resuscitation area. The resuscitation trolley should have sides to minimise convection in the immediate vicinity of the baby.

Evaporative losses

The wet newborn loses large amounts of heat very rapidly by this route; he should therefore be dried all over, including his head and scalp, as soon as possible after delivery, preferably with warm towels, to eliminate conductive loss.

Radiant losses

Heat is lost by radiation onto the nearest solid objects which, for example, in the case of single glazed windows in winter can be very cold indeed. For this reason, the infant should be covered (again including his head), ideally with the warm towels alluded to above. Should active resuscitation be required as much of the baby as possible should be covered, since when the baby is asphyxiated he is not able to produce any heat himself, and he will therefore cool down even more rapidly.

It should be remembered that babies at birth have a temperature 0.5–1°C higher than their mothers. Sadly, it is not uncommon for even normal, healthy, full term babies to drop their body temperature to 35–35.5°C by 15–30 minutes of age due to slipshod care in the labour ward. The labour ward may not have been warm enough, there may have been draughts (a particular horror is air-conditioning vents near resuscitation trolleys), or those responsible for his care did not dry him or cover him up soon enough after birth. Most neonatal illnesses, in particular lung disorders, hypoglycaemia and coagulation disorders are more likely to occur and be more severe if the baby is allowed to get cold.

The problem is entirely preventable by attention to detail: before the delivery, close all doors and windows in the delivery room, and turn off all air circulation systems likely to blast over the baby. The temperature of the room should be at least 20°C, higher if a pre-term infant is anticipated. The resuscitation trolley, with its overhead radiant heater switched on, should be put in the warmest and least draughty part of the room. As soon as the infant is delivered, he should be placed on pre-warmed towels, dried in them and then wrapped and swaddled in them.

Anything that involves leaving the baby naked for more than a few seconds such as bathing (p. 78) or various fashionable components of early mother–baby skin–skin contact should only be done in warm rooms (23–25°C) or under a radiant heat source.

CORD CLAMPING

The time at which the cord should be clamped after delivery is a subject which generates violent passions quite unnecessarily. Once the baby is delivered, there is no point delaying cord clamping since it merely allows the naked infant to cool off. The dangers to a neonate of missing out on his placental transfusion are overestimated particularly if he is normal and term. For ill or pre-term infants the priority is to get them to the resuscitaire as soon as possible, and if they are found to be hypotensive subsequently, this can be treated easily by transfusion. Furthermore, giving a large placental transfusion, and making the baby polycythaemic, increases the incidence of many neonatal conditions including transient tachypnoea, jaundice, hypoglycaemia, seizures and heart failure.

It is of course essential that there is an entirely foolproof routine for clamping or ligating the umbilical cord in the labour ward, otherwise a fatal neonatal haemorrhage can ensue.

CORD CARE

Correct care of the umbilical cord and stump during the first week significantly reduces the incidence of infection in the neonate. The necrotic tissue of the dying Wharton's jelly is readily colonised by pathogenic organisms from the environment which may spread to cause skin, conjunctival or systemic infection in the baby, or breast infection in the mother. Various techniques have been used to prevent this, but I prefer spraying the umbilical cord with an antibiotic powder such as Polybactrin (Elias Jones, 1986). Although in very small babies repeated use of such sprays has resulted in the transepidermal absorption of toxic levels of antibiotics, this is not a hazard with single use, or in mature babies with a thick normally keratinised skin. Spraying the umbilical cord with antibiotic is of particular importance in an infant in whom it is likely that umbilical vessel catheterisation will be needed, since this lessens the likelihood of having to pass the catheter through a contaminated field. The cord must always be sprayed before the umbilical clamp or ligature is applied. Good cord care is, of course, particularly important in developing countries where neonatal tetanus gains access by this route.

LABELLING

A tag bearing the baby's/mother's name must be securely attached to his wrist or ankle in the labour ward, care being taken to fit it such that it is neither too tight nor will slip off. Increasingly, security devices may need to be incorporated into these tags. Only with meticulous attention to these apparently trivial details can the horrors of baby swapping or snatching be prevented.

EYE PROPHYLAXIS

In many countries, but not in the UK, it is routine to instil one drop of 0.5 per cent $AgNO_3$ into each eye immediately after delivery to prevent gonococcal ophthalmia. The technique is effective, but causes an irritant chemical conjunctivitis in up to 90 per cent of babies (Nishida and Risenberg, 1975). Whether or not it is justified depends on the incidence of gonorrhoea in the local population of pregnant women.

VITAMIN K

Haemorrhagic disease of the newborn is a potentially serious condition affecting approximately 1:400 live births. It is more likely to occur in breast-fed infants, infants delivered instrumentally particularly if they were asphyxiated, pre-term babies, infants of mothers taking anticonvulsants and aspirin (pp. 20–21, 36), and for reasons that are not understood, black babies.

The condition exists in two forms, classical early haemorrhagic disease occurring within the first week in which bleeding occurs from the gut, cord stump or following minor surgery such as circumcision. Late haemorrhagic disease develops around one month of age, and as well as peripheral haemorrhage, intra-cerebral haemorrhage often develops. Late haemorrhagic disease is most common in breast-fed babies or those with underlying liver disease.

Both forms of the disease can be prevented in all neonates by appropriate vitamin K prophylaxis after delivery, but this therapy has become extremely controversial in recent years. In the mid-1980s it was suggested that any vitamin K prophylaxis was unnecessary, but this unwise advice was soon scotched by an epidemic of the vitamin K-deficient intracerebral haemorrhages.

In the 1990s, studies from Bristol, about which there are considerable methodological anxieties, suggested that i.m. vitamin K after birth increased the incidence of leukaemia in later childhood, but several larger subsequent studies have failed to confirm this association. I believe, therefore, that all babies should receive 1 mg of i.m. vitamin K at birth. This prevents all early (classical) and late haemorrhagic disease. No oral preparation licensed for neonatal use exists at present in the UK, though Konakion mixed micelles (Konakion MM), at present available for adult use, may soon be licensed for the neonate. Until that time, for those not prepared to give i.m. vitamin K to babies the only alternative which will sustain adequate coagulation and prevent late HDN is 1–2 mg of the i.m. preparation of vitamin K given orally immediately after delivery followed by a further 0.5 mg on two occasions during the first month (Rennie and Kelsall, 1994).

Refusal to give vitamin K to the baby gives him about a 1:1000 chance of developing haemorrhagic disease of the newborn of any type, and a 1:10 000 chance of developing an intracerebral bleed due to this preventable condition.

BATHING

It is steeped (*sic*) in the arcane mysteries of midwifery that a newborn baby should be bathed immediately after delivery to remove all the nasty things he is covered in like blood, vernix, meconium, hibitane cream, Polybactrin and so on! This is nonsense, and is one of the most common causes of neonatal hypothermia; furthermore, it snatches the baby away from his parents at a time then they want to enjoy him. Bathing babies in labour wards should be forbidden.

MEASUREMENT

Babies should always be weighed after birth – apart from anything else weight and sex are the two things parents always want to know before ringing the grandparents.

Routine length measurements are not necessary. Stretching a tape measure alongside a supine infant, or dangling one alongside the neonate held upside down by his ankles is so inaccurate as to be meaningless. If it is believed that length is an important measurement it should be done properly and carefully with an infant stadiometer, taking care to have the baby properly extended (Fig. 5.1).

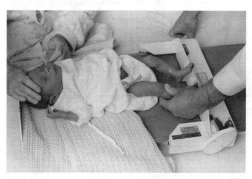

FIGURE 5.1 Infant stadiometer in use. Note the need to hold the baby's legs straight.

BONDING

(Richards, 1992)

Although it is now clear that denying a baby access to his mother in the first hour of life will not condemn them both to a life of mutual emotional incompatibility, three facts are very clear. The first is that the mother has waited 9 months to have her baby, and now she has got him she and the father should be allowed to love him and enjoy him; the second is that babies (unless drugged by injudicious use of narcotic analgesics just before delivery) are particularly alert, bright eyed and appealing in the first 30–60 minutes after delivery; and the third is that putting the baby to the breast at this time is an important determinant of successful long-term lactation, p. 144).

In making arrangements for families and babies to be together immediately after delivery there is, however, no need to be kinky with everyone naked, in the dark or under water! Indeed from the point of view of the baby's temperature such activities can be very dangerous (see above). The snugly swaddled neonate should be given to his parents as soon after delivery as possible. If they so wish, the parents and their child should then be left to enjoy their first hour together in a warm and pleasantly lit room, with the mother in a comfortable bed big enough for the baby to lie beside her and breast-feed. If the mother wants help in putting the baby to the breast it should be given; otherwise the professionals should keep out.

REFERENCES

Elias Jones, A.C. (1986). Triple antibiotic spray application to umbilical cord. *Early Human Development* **13**, 299–302.

Nishida, H. and Risenberg, H.M. (1975). Silver nitrate ophthalmic solution and chemical conjunctivitis. *Pediatrics* **56**, 368–373.

Rennie, J-M. and Kelsall, A.W.R. (1994). Vitamin K prophylaxis in the newborn – again. *Archives of Disease in Childhood* **70**, 248–251.

Richards, M.P.M. (1992). Bonding. In: Psychological aspects of neonatal care. In: *Textbook of Neonatology*. Ed. Roberton, N.R.C. Churchill Livingstone, 2nd Edn. London, Edinburgh, pp. 29–42.

Rutter, N. (1992). Temperature control and its disorders. In: *Textbook of Neonatology*. Ed. Roberton, N.R.C. Churchill Livingstone, 2nd Ed. London, Edinburgh, pp. 217–231.

6

ROUTINE POSTNATAL CARE

Examining (Chapter 7), screening (Chapter 8) and feeding (Chapter 9) normal babies is described in detail elsewhere.

HOME VERSUS HOSPITAL

It has been recognised for many years that the major perinatal risk to mother and baby occurs in the few hours on each side of delivery. As a result, many women having produced a bouncy normal baby with a good Apgar go home within 12 hours. The management outlined in the rest of this chapter applies to home as well as the postnatal ward.

ADMISSION ROUTINE

On arrival in a postnatal ward (PNW) from the labour ward, the baby should have his temperature, pulse and respiration recorded. Thereafter, pulse and respiration should be recorded twice daily, and temperature daily, though it is arguable whether more harm is done by stuffing thermometers up infants' back passages than good is done by identifying hypothermia or pyrexia before other signs are present and there is certainly no need to do it to well babies in their own homes.

ROOMING-IN

The standard management in hospital should be that the mother can have her baby with her in a cot beside her bed whenever she wishes – throughout the 24 hours if necessary – the practice of 'rooming-in'. In this way she can learn to respond to and manage his every demand and need. If she is ill, and still in hospital, or if she requests it, the baby can go into the ward nursery overnight. However, if the baby is in the nursery overnight the mother should always be asked if she wishes to be woken to feed him.

Feeding should be on a demand basis only (pp. 142–3) and this is infinitely easier to manage if the baby is in a cot beside his mother.

SLEEPING POSITION

Much recent data suggests that the risk of sudden infant death syndrome is less in babies sleeping on their back or side. This practice should be started on the postnatal ward.

THE NORMAL NEONATE

CARDIORESPIRATORY FUNCTION

The normal term infant has a pulse rate of 110–160, and a blood pressure of 55/30–80/50; sinus arrhythmia is rare. His respiratory rate is 30–60/minute without any apnoeic attacks, though during rapid eye movement (REM) sleep his breathing is often irregular with pauses of 3–5 seconds. In non-REM sleep his breathing is very regular and shallow. When awake, aroused or hungry, the pulse rate and respiratory rate may rise to 180/minute and 60/minute respectively. Some postmature babies may have a normal pulse rate of 80–90/minute when asleep.

TEMPERATURE CONTROL

The term baby usually maintains his temperature very accurately around 37°C so that any departure from this always demands careful evaluation, in particular, to exclude sepsis (p. 293). For the standard, healthy, term baby who is clothed and kept in a cot, keeping his bedroom or the postnatal wards at a temperature of 20–22°C is adequate. If the room temperature falls below 20°C, the baby should always wear a hat, and be swaddled with 1–2 blankets. It is very important, however, not to overheat the baby by over-wrapping him, lying him by a radiator, putting him in direct sunlight, or putting some external heat source in a cot with him.

WEIGHT CHANGES

After weighing a baby at birth, there is little point weighing him again until the third or fourth day, since all babies lose weight during this time, primarily due to water loss from the extracellular fluid. Thereafter, from the fourth or fifth day he should be weighed daily or every other day until he is gaining weight consistently, as this is the most effective check that the feeding, by breast or bottle, is going well.

The weight loss in the first few days should not exceed 10 per cent of his birthweight, and should always be assessed in relative terms, even though it means that a 4.50 kg baby may lose 450 g (i.e. 1 lb) in the first 5 days. From this age onwards the normal baby should gain weight at about 30 g/day until the age of 6 months.

URINE OUTPUT

Many neonates pass urine immediately after birth and regularly thereafter. Others, particularly if breast-fed with a poor fluid intake, may pass very little urine in the first 24–36 hours. Thereafter they pass 40–60 ml of urine/kg/24 hours, usually when they are fed or when their perineum is exposed to fresh air. It is exceptionally unusual for any illness to present in an otherwise normal baby with just anuria or oliguria.

BOWEL ACTIVITY

As with urine, many babies defecate in the first 2 minutes, and usually regularly thereafter. Initially they pass meconium, a dark greenish compound which is composed of intestinal secretions, bile, including bilirubin, swallowed amniotic debris and the remains of desquamated intestinal mucosal cells. After 2 or 3 days 'changing' stools, a mixture of meconium and more normal stools are passed, and once feeding is well established the stools change completely to a normal colour. Breast-fed babies pass very soft, mustardy-yellow stools, often with every feed, and their stools are acid. Bottle-fed babies pass a less acid stool (p. 125) which is usually firmer and paler in colour. They often pass only one or two stools per day.

The bacterial flora in both breast-fed and bottle-fed babies consists of enterobacteriaceae (such as *E. coli*), enterococci, bacteroides and bifidobacteria (lactobacillus), but the latter are present in larger numbers, and are the predominant organism in breast-fed babies.

PREVENTION OF INFECTION ON A POSTNATAL WARD

HAND WASHING

The major risk to the baby is from the medical and nursing staff (p. 217), who even on a routine PNW must be meticulous in washing their hands before they touch or handle any babies. One of the advantages of being at home is avoiding these cross infection hazards, but even there the family in the first few weeks should wash their hands before doing anything to the baby. The details of preventing cross infection are outlined in Chapter 16.

CORD CARE

If the cord has been properly treated in the labour ward (p. 75), it should not become infected in the next few days, and this also helps to keep down the general level of infection. However, if it does look as though the umbilical stump is becoming infected further daily spraying with antibiotic powder should be started (p. 222). Good cord care means that the cord stays dry and does not drop off. This upsets senior midwives and mothers-in-law who feel that this is an unnatural happening. To allay their anxieties, it is our habit to cut off the redundant Wharton's jelly, level with the anterior abdominal wall, on the fourth or fifth day.

VISITORS

Healthy visitors are not an infectious hazard, and the number a mother and her baby are allowed should be decided on a common sense basis. If every family member in an extended family wanted to visit often and at length it would not only exhaust the mother and the baby, but would create chaos in an open ward. Other patients can do without relatives of the patient in the next bed trampling all over them and theirs! However, grandparents, husbands and siblings should be allowed very free access to the new family member as indeed happens at home!

Unhealthy visitors should in general stay away, following the guidelines in Table 3.2 if access is deemed important (e.g. fathers).

FATE OF THE FORESKIN

Circumcision of either sex in the neonatal period should be seen for what it is – a tribal ritual. It is never indicated medically, and therefore should not be carried out.

For those who elect to have their child treated in this way the medical profession should remind them that the parts in question are not bereft of nerve endings and contain blood vessels. Adequate analgesia and vitamin K should therefore be provided.

All neonatal males have 'phimosis'; the foreskin is not meant to be retractile at this age, and the parents must be told to leave it alone and not to try and retract it. Forcible retraction in infancy tears the tissues at the tip of the foreskin causing scarring, and is the most common cause of genuine phimosis later in life.

WELL BABY CARE

Since the baby was not bathed in the labour ward, he should probably be washed during the second or third day. The first wash can be just 'topping and tailing' – that is, washing his face and hair, and cleaning up his groins and perineum. For primiparae this first bath may need to be a supervised or even demonstrated affair. One of the major purposes of the inpatient postnatal stay is to reinforce the mothercraft classes which the mother, hopefully, attended during her pregnancy, so that she goes home confident in her ability to care for her baby, and in particular feed him, keep him warm, bathe him, change his nappies and dress him. Although these remarks may seem banal, it is surprising in 1996 how inexperienced and unconfident are many young women raised in small nuclear families and with no exposure to child rearing until they themselves are expected to do it.

7

EXAMINATION OF THE NEWBORN

—

GENERAL PRINCIPLES

Newborn babies are examined in two situations, firstly, when they are ill, when the examination is carried out to evaluate the presenting symptoms, and, secondly, on a routine basis as a screening procedure some time in the early neonatal period. The aims of the two examinations are clearly different, though the general principles of the examination are much the same.

It has to be recognised, however, that there are considerable limitations to the formal clinical examination of a very small person. He cannot localise pain, or describe his symptoms. Picking up subtleties of air entry or bronchial breathing is not possible in the 800 g infant's chest; interpreting the second heart sound when the heart is beating 180 times per minute is beyond the auditory acuity of most paediatricians, and sophisticated CNS examination is impossible in a patient not capable of doing the finger–nose test or assessing which way his toe is pointing. All these problems are magnified if the baby decides not to cooperate with the clinician by howling and thrashing around.

It is impossible, therefore, to exclude clinically many serious diseases such as meningitis, pneumothorax or pyelonephritis which would give clear signs and symptoms in older children and adults. Recourse to laboratory or radiological investigation is therefore often required to evaluate clinical problems in non-specifically ill neonates (p. 297). Conversely, the neonatal clinician must learn to interpret subtle signs indicating deterioration. 'Not liking the look of' a baby is a very important physical sign which should never be ignored.

The clinician should also learn all the tricks that will enable him to achieve the maximum from the examination. Take time, and use the experts (nurses, mother) to undress the baby. A baby is calmest when being fed, so learn to examine him fully while he is sucking at the breast. Never startle him with a cold stethoscope, a cold environment or sudden movements. Listen to the heart with a warm stethoscope at the start of the examination – since the baby may never be quiet again! Leave things that are bound to upset him till last. These include taking the blood pressure, prizing open his mouth and eyes, putting a tape measure round his head, checking his hips (pp. 101–4), doing a rectal examination, and, of course, examining an inflamed or injured area. Be an opportunist: if the baby has his bowels open or passes urine, are the products normal and produced normally? If he has his eyes open, look at them; if a fractious baby howls and thrashes about, have a good look in his mouth and note if his facial and limb movements are normal and symmetrical. In general, though, it is fruitless to examine a fractious baby and he should be calmed down by a feed, or by sucking a dummy or the examiner's finger.

SYSTEMATIC EVALUATION

The examination outlined in the following pages is that indicated in an ill baby, or in a baby found to have a problem on the routine neonatal clinical examination (p. 106) which is a procedure designed to identify covert problems in an asymptomatic patient.

GENERAL APPEARANCE

Standing back and having a good long look at the baby is the first, and often most useful, part of all paediatric examinations, never mind the neonatal one. At the end of this preliminary scrutiny, the examiner should have decided whether the baby looks ill or not. Important components of this assessment include:

- Is the baby cyanosed?
- Is the baby jaundiced?
- Is the baby well perfused or not, i.e. are his peripheries pink; is his skin a homogeneous pink colour without any mottling or easily visible superficial veins; is capillary filling rapid?
- Does he look pink enough: pallor may mean shock, acidaemia or anaemia?
- Are there any skin rashes; is he meconium stained?
- Is his posture normal; does he move all parts of his body including his face, or not; if he is moving them, are the movements normal and symmetrical, or does he have fits?
- Does he look normal facially, or is he a 'syndrome', i.e. does he look like Down's syndrome?
- If his eyes are open, do they move normally, are the pupils equal and are any opacities visible in the cornea or lens?
- Is his respiration present! and normal in rate (< 40/minute) and pattern?
- Are there any lumps, bumps or swellings, inflamed or otherwise, visible in the position he has adopted (do not move him at this stage)?
- Is there abdominal distension, with or without visible peristalsis or areas of redness?
- Look at the sheets round the baby; are they covered with vomit, urine, blood or faeces and, if so, what sort?

At the end of this period of perusal, the clinician should have a pretty good provisional idea of what is going on in a symptomatic baby, and can proceed to a systematic examination, remembering to grasp any opportunity that presents itself. As well as this general perusal of the infant, it is worth remembering three general facts about examining newborn babies:

- Certain groups of babies, in particular small-for-dates neonates, infants of diabetic mothers and twins have an increased incidence of malformations, though probably only 2–3 times the average.
- The presence of one abnormality, no matter how small, e.g. a single transverse palmar crease, should alert the examiner to search for other malformations.
- In the presence of more than three or four minor malformations (or major ones for that matter) consider doing a karyotype and also obtain a photograph of the baby so that changes in his appearance can be carefully documented.

CARDIOVASCULAR EXAMINATION

The normal baby should be pink with a heart rate usually between 110 and 160, and a blood pressure of 55/30–80/50. Any suspicion of central cyanosis demands confirmation by blood gas analysis, and if present further investigation by CXR, ECG and echocardiogram.

Particularly in large, sleeping, term babies the pulse rate may be as low as 80–90, but anything lower than this, even if asymptomatic, should be checked by ECG. Rates above 160/minute at rest and with a normal temperature usually indicate some underlying problem including heart disease, sepsis or lung disease. The child should be investigated accordingly. Very fast rates – greater than 180–200/minute – are difficult to count accurately and can be >300/minute. Such infants should always have their heart rate checked by ECG, and be investigated further.

The peripheral pulses must be examined, and to exclude coarctation of the aorta the femoral pulses *must always* be checked to confirm that they are of normal volume and synchronous with the radial pulses.

Femoral pulses can be very difficult to feel in the first 24–48 hours of life, particularly in a fat, vigorous 4.00 kg baby with vernix besmeared groins. In such cases, the baby's pulses should be re-examined a day or two later (unless he has other signs of coarctation such as a murmur or heart failure), when they will usually be easily palpable. If there is any doubt about the pulses, the blood pressure in the arms and legs should be checked.

Isolated abnormalities of blood pressure are rarely detected, since, apart from anything else, it is usually only in symptomatic babies that anyone goes to the bother of measuring it. In the first few days, as closure of the ductus distorts the aortic isthmus, the leg blood pressures may be up to 15–20 mmHg lower than the arm without the presence of coarctation (deSwiet *et al.*, 1974). A sustained systolic blood pressure above 100 mmHg in a neonate is always abnormal and justifies investigation.

Listen to the first and second heart sounds; S_2 may normally stay single up to 48 hours of age. However, detecting subtle nuances of the heart sounds, or ejection clicks in a baby with a heart rate of > 160/minute is strictly for the professionals.

When talking about the murmurs in the neonatal period, five important facts must be remembered:
- Up to 60–80 per cent of all neonates have a murmur in the first 24–48 hours of life. It is usually Grade 1–2/6 and mid-systolic.
- Lone diastolic murmurs in the neonate are staggeringly rare, i.e. all murmurs are either systolic or systolic plus diastolic.
- The vast majority (>95 per cent) of babies with murmurs in the first few days of life either do not

have heart disease or have a defect that will recover spontaneously (e.g. small VSD or a PDA).

- Many infants with serious CHD do not have murmurs in the first few days, though they may have subtle changes in their heart sounds and pulses, or be cyanosed.
- A loud systolic murmur may be due to an extra-cardiac shunt, such as an arterio-venous malformation, characteristically in the liver or brain.

The management of the child with a murmur is outlined on p. 260.

EXAMINATION OF THE RESPIRATORY SYSTEM

The normal neonate breathes 35–45/minute without any evidence of distress. He has good air entry on auscultation, and both inspiration and expiration are audible.

The presence of intrapulmonary pathology can usually be detected simply by looking at the baby.

- He will be tachypnoeic, apnoeic, dyspnoeic or blue. If these features are absent, the baby can be assumed to have normal lungs and further clinical examination is unnecessary. However, if these suggestive clinical features are present, the following points should always be noted before proceeding to a CXR.
- Listening to the chest and hearing crackles and wheezes confirms that the baby has a lung problem!
- Dullness to percussion is rarely detected in a supine baby, but if present may indicate a very large pleural effusion. Dullness may also indicate collapse or consolidation but is only found with gross abnormalities; the absence of this physical sign is thus of no value in excluding lung pathology.
- Increased resonance on percussion, and a bulging chest on one side may be present if there is a pneumothorax, and if this is large and under

tension a mediastinal shift may be detected; there may also be abdominal distension secondary to the diaphragm being depressed by the intra-pleural air under pressure. A pneumothorax will always cause the non-specific dyspnoea and tachyp-noea of intra-thoracic mischief, and can only be excluded by CXR.

- Decreased air entry is a feature of many forms of severe neonatal lung disease such as RDS. It is never found without concurrent respiratory diffi-culty, and its main value is in identifying the side of the lesion in unilateral problems such as pneu-mothorax or lung collapse.

- Bowel sounds in the chest in a mildly dyspnoeic infant indicate a diaphragmatic hernia, but this condition usually presents with marked respiratory distress immediately after delivery.

EXAMINATION OF THE UPPER RESPIRATORY TRACT

ENT disease (other than malformations) is rare in the neonate. Stridor may be seen if the larynx has been damaged by intubation, or if there is a con-genital laryngeal problem. However, this is rare. Even rarer is an obstructed breathing pattern noted only when the infant's mouth is closed; this characteristi-cally suggests nasal obstruction (choanal atresia), and this diagnosis should be established by trying to pass a nasal catheter through each nostril.

In a non-specifically unwell and febrile older neonate, particularly one who has a cleft palate or an indwelling endotracheal tube (both of which com-promise Eustachian tube function), otitis media should be considered, and the ear examined oto-scopically. The tympanic membrane is more difficult to see than in older children because of its more oblique, downward-facing position, but if seen to be injected, it means infection.

EXAMINATION OF THE ABDOMEN AND ALIMENTARY TRACT

Always look in a baby's mouth. Teeth may be present, as may ranulae (cysts in the floor of the mouth). An abnormality of the tongue or palate is easily missed, in particular a small posterior mid-line cleft palate.

The liver may be palpable 2 cm below the right costal margin in normal babies, and in 15 per cent of normal babies 1–2 cm of spleen may be felt. If either organ is bigger than this, further investigation is necessary, particularly if there is jaundice (suggesting infection, either a primary hepatitis or a non-specific response to infection), dyspnoea (suggesting heart failure or a pneumothorax – see above), purpura/petechiae (suggesting infection, congenital or otherwise), pallor (suggesting a haemolytic anaemia), or the enlargement is gross (suggesting any of the above plus an inborn metabolic error or storage disease). The kidneys, particularly the left one, can often be palpated in normal babies. Enlarged kidneys require investigation, usually in the first place by ultrasound. Renal enlargement can be a non-specific sign of septicaemia (not necessarily due to urinary infection), but can also be due to urinary tract obstruction, hydronephrosis, some form of cystic disease, renal tumours or renal vein thrombosis, and a palpable kidney can be due to it being displaced downwards by an adrenal mass.

The assessment of the baby with antenatal ultrasound diagnosis of urinary tract abnormalities is outlined on p. 306. Always examine male babies carefully to exclude a large bladder since this may be the only sign of posterior urethral valves which always need urgent treatment. An important co-existing physical sign is whether the baby can pass urine in a good stream. However, whether or not that physical sign is present, a persistently enlarged bladder must always be investigated by ultrasound and probably by cystography.

Enlargement of all intra-abdominal organs, plus the presence of an intra-abdominal mass (e.g. a cyst or a tumour, both exceptionally rare), will of course cause abdominal distension. The differential diagnosis of other causes of a distended belly is discussed on p. 299.

It is always recommended that the umbilicus should be examined. However, in the absence of symptoms little is to be gained from this exercise. If it is infected, red and discharging, this should be treated (p. 222). When the cord separates, or it is cut off, there is often a small ooze of blood which responds to local pressure. Discharge of clear fluid from the umbilicus can, in exceptionally rare circumstances, be urine from a patent urachus. Malformations of the umbilicus, e.g. omphalocoele, are howlingly obvious, and the number of blood vessels present is really only of interest to those who need to catheterize them. Contrary to popular belief, the presence of only two blood vessels (i.e. one artery and one vein) is of no significance in a baby with no other abnormalities on clinical examination. Granuloma of the cord is dealt with on p. 269.

Examining the anus, other than confirming that it is there, is rarely of value. If a baby is bleeding PR (p. 265) the anal margin should be examined for a fissure, and occasionally it is worth attempting a 'proctoscopy' using an otoscope. Rectal examination should only be done in the presence of intra-abdominal pathology; it is not indicated as a routine.

NEUROLOGICAL EXAMINATION

By far and away the most useful part of the neurological examination is watching the naked baby, his posture, his face and his movements. It must be stressed that the neonate does not show signs of meningism, and the diagnosis of meningitis can only be excluded by a lumbar puncture carried out in response to the non-specific signs of infection (pp. 294–6).

Fits in the neonate, particularly the premature one, may be much more subtle than in older infants. The fit may be little more than an apnoeic attack, some minor movements of the mouth or eyes, or unusual limb movements, and will only be noticed by carefully scrutinising the baby. Typical tonic-clonic fits are unusual.

In no other part of the examination is it more important to have the baby in the ideal state.

The behavioural state of the newborn has been divided in to five stages:

- I asleep – quiet sleep (non-REM)
- II asleep – active (REM)
- III awake: quiet
- IV awake: active
- V crying

For most parts of the neurological examination the baby needs to be in stage III, since in IV and V he is unexaminable and in stage I and II it is not only impossible to test many activities, e.g. vision, but in stage II, for example, much reflex activity is centrally inhibited.

After observing the baby, check his spine and skull for overlying cutaneous lesions (e.g. haemangiomas) or dermal sinuses which could communicate with the theca (NB a sacrococcygeal pit is normal, p. 274); also, check the spine for kyphosis or scoliosis.

Always measure the size of the baby's head; the occipto-frontal circumference (OFC) is measured by putting the tape measure over the occipital protruberance and round the frontal bones just below the hair line. This is fine in a normal-shaped head since it is the maximum circumference, but in an abnormal-shaped head the maximum circumference should always be sought since this is the only measurement which is reproducible.

Check the fontanelles – the anterior should not normally be more than 4 × 3 cm, and the posterior 1 × 1 cm. Examine the sutures which should be < 1 cm wide and check if there is an expansion of the suture line between the anterior fontanelle and the posterior fontanelle. This so-called third fontanelle is a feature of Down's syndrome. When interpreting the suture and fontanelle size, it is essential to know the OFC and if this is normal having wide sutures or a wide fontanelle is usually normal. However, if the OFC is above the 97th centile or grossly disproportionate compared with the rest of the baby, then hydrocephalus is likely.

The skull bones often overlap in the neonatal period, giving a 'step-up' feeling as the examiner's finger moves from one side to another, and a 'step-down' feeling when moving in the opposite direction. A ridge along the suture, i.e. a step-up in both directions, is abnormal; this suggests craniostenosis and merits further investigation by skull X-ray and ultrasound.

Transillumination of the head may show up abnormal intracranial collections of fluid, but the ready availability of cranial ultrasound in most hospitals has rendered this investigation almost obsolete in the neonate.

Tone and power should be assessed. Tone can be checked by doing the traction response (Fig. 7.1), or by ventral suspension (Fig. 7.2), by passively moving and shaking a limb or, as always, by just looking. For example, does the baby's mouth always hang open? Although professional neonatal neurologists read a great deal into subtle alterations in tone, I believe that it is a very difficult and subjective physical sign to interpret. Basically, all one can usually do is to assess whether the tone is within the normal range, or whether the baby is like a rag doll or pretty rigid, both

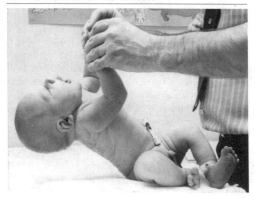

FIGURE 7.1 The normal traction response.

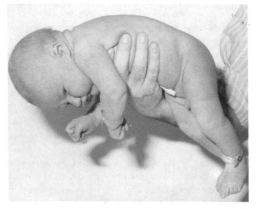

FIGURE 7.2 The normal ventral suspension position — adopted by a term neonate with normal tone.

of which suggest serious underlying CNS problems.

Power is assessed best by watching the baby and seeing whether he can raise his limbs against gravity, or watching to see how he moves his head when lying prone. Coordination is impossible to test, and testing sensation means doing something nasty to the baby like pinching or pricking him and seeing if he responds.

The conventional tendon reflexes are present in the term neonate, but the plantar response is usually extensor.

Sphincter function should always be assessed, noting how the baby passes urine and whether his anus is patulous.

Most of the cranial nerves can be tested.

- I   Not possible.
- II   The newborn can see. The most effective way of checking this is to have him alert and looking at the examiner's face, which he will follow when it is moved from side to side. Examining the eyes, cornea, pupils and sclera can be done at the same time. A cataract may be noted as a white spot in the pupil. However, unless there is a family history of cataract, or the infant has other signs of a disease in which cataract is present, there is no point in routinely examining all babies for this condition. If ophthalmoscopic examination is indicated it is probably a waste of time to attempt it without instilling mydriatic drops, and without the baby having his eyes open spontaneously, ideally during a feed. Forcing open a baby's eye lids is doomed to failure. If accurate ophthalmoscopy is necessary, examination under anaesthetic is justified.
- III,IV,VI Ocular position, pupillary response, and external ocular movements can be assessed when checking the visual function.
- V,VII   These are best tested by watching the baby's face during sucking and crying.
- VIII   *Vestibular.* This can be tested by swinging

the baby round the examiner to evoke rotatory nystagmus. The startled neonate usually demonstrates this physical sign when he opens his eyes in amazement at his treatment shortly before he howls in protest.

Auditory: Routine screening of all babies for deafness is not yet justified. However, if there is any clinical suspicion about a baby's response to sound, malformations of the ear, a family history of deafness or any neonatal condition likely to cause deafness such as severe jaundice or meningitis, the baby should be carefully assessed in an auditory response cradle, or by using one of the newer electrophysiological tests.

• IX–XII If the baby can suck and swallow normally, these nerves are working. The palate can usually be seen to move normally as can the tongue. Fasciculation of the tongue is a useful early sign of Werdnig–Hoffman disease in the floppy neonate.

Many automatisms, such as the grasp response, the Moro response,* and walking responses can be elicited in the normal neonate. They add precious little, if anything, to what has been learned by watching the baby's spontaneous movements. Although the presence of an Erb's palsy (pp. 253–5) is highlighted by an asymmetrical Moro, the lesion should be detected earlier by simple observation, without the need to shake the poor baby about.

---

*This response is elicited by startling the neonate, or suddenly extending his neck. This results in his eyes opening, his arms being fully abducted and extended, and his fingers extended, followed by his arms and fingers flexing and abducting.

EXAMINATION OF LIMBS, FACE AND SKELETAL SYSTEM

This is by and large a matter of simple observation. Is there a limb on each corner with the normal five digits connected to it? Are the limbs, joints and digits normal in shape, size and range of movement? Abnormalities of limb movement suggest neurological lesions, fracture or the pseudoparalysis of arthritis or osteomyelitis.

Are all the facial features present and normal? Odd looking children should be checked in the syndrome atlases (Chapter 20).

By convention we look carefully at the baby's hands to look for things like single palmar creases, or clinodactyly (a curved little finger), though if any of these are present as isolated findings, they are usually inconsequential, and if they are features of Down's syndrome, that diagnosis should have been made on a gestält basis.

The skull and axial skeleton is examined as part of the CNS examination.

Many lumps and bumps may be detected on physical examination in addition to those noted at the original superficial scrutiny. Their nature (p. 272) should always be explained to the mother, and their management outlined.

The single most important part of the examination of the skeletal system, and indeed of the routine neonatal clinical examination, is the examination for congenital dislocation of the hip.

The neonatal hip examination is carried out in two stages, and must be done with the infant relaxed and not struggling, ideally in states I–III (p. 96). Firstly, the thighs are held as shown in Fig. 7.3(a). They are then fully abducted. If the legs can be made to lie flat as shown, the hips are not dislocated. During the movement of the legs to the fully abducted position, a dislocated femoral head may be felt to 'clunk' back into the acetabulum. This is Ortolani's sign and indicates a dislocated hip. It is crucial to ensure that the hip abducts fully. If it does not do so, it may be because, despite careful manipulation and trying to pull the femur away from the acetabulum during Ortolani's manoeuvre, the femoral head will not disengage from its dislocated position. The thigh will then only move to 45° from the vertical, and not the full 90°. This is the type of CDH that is most easy to miss on examination.

In the second phase of the examination the leg is returned to the position in Fig. 7.3(b). While simul-

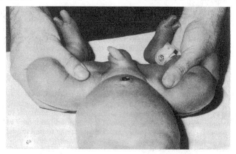

FIGURE 7.3(a) Clinical examination to exclude CDH. The thighs are fully abducted while held in the grip depicted. If the leg can be made to lie flat as shown in Fig. 7.3(a), the hip is not dislocated. The dislocated femoral head may clunk into the acetabulum during this manoeuvre (Ortolani's sign). It is very important to make sure that the hip fully abducts. Failure to do so may be because the hip is dislocated and fails to reduce during Ortolani's manoeuvre; the hip will then stay at 45° from the horizontal. This is the type of CDH which is most easy to miss on examination.

taneously applying lateral traction to pull the femur away from the acetabulum, the examiner presses downwards and outwards with his thumbs to try to push the femoral head out of the acetabulum. If the hip dislocates (and this is in fact painless), this is a positive Barlow's sign, and it is always possible to flip the femoral head back into the acetabulum by doing Ortolani's manoeuvre. In some patients, when doing Barlow's manoeuvre, the femoral head is clearly unstable within the acetabulum and rattles around within it without ever dislocating. This is also a significant finding and should be noted.

A variety of creaking and clicking noises can be produced during the Barlow manoeuvre, in particular. It is doubtful if these are of significance.

The main problem, however, with the Ortolani and

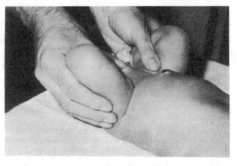

FIGURE 7.3(b) The legs are then returned to the position in Fig. 7.3(b) while simultaneously applying lateral traction to pull the femoral head out of the acetabulum and pressing downwards with the thumbs to push the femoral head back out of the joint. If the hip dislocates, this is a positive Barlow's sign and it is usually very easy to flip the femoral head back into position by doing Ortolani's manoeuvre. If during Barlow's manoeuvre the femoral head is very loose in the acetabulum, but does not actually dislocate over the lip of the acetabulum, it should probably be treated like CDH.

Barlow procedures is that they have a very poor specificity and sensitivity. Despite their use, many cases of CDH are missed, and excessive use of the Barlow's test may even increase hip instability (Moore, 1989). More important, the majority of hips found to be abnormal on Barlow's test become stable and normal within a few days and do not require any treatment.

To try to improve diagnostic accuracy and efficiency, ultrasound assessment of the hip joint is indicated in the neonatal period. There is as yet no place for *routine* ultrasound examination of *all* hips. However to reduce the number of cases missed, in addition to doing the Ortolani and Barlow manoeuvres, ultrasound scanning should be done on the hips of all at-risk babies – those delivered by the breech, or who have a limb or spine deformity such as meningomyelocoele or talipes, or who have a family history of CDH.

In addition, those with an abnormal Barlow or Ortolani sign should be ultrasounded, including those with 'clicking' hips. Only those with definite ultrasound abnormalities by, say, two weeks of age need splinting (Clarke, 1994), sparing many babies the inconvenience, discomfort and possible hip injury from splinting (pp. 313–5).

GENITALIA

Ambiguous genitalia require urgent clinical and biochemical assessment (p. 318), though in most cases this can be initiated with the baby on the postnatal ward with its mother. Serious abnormalities of the external genitalia in the female are rare; a skin tag at the fourchette is common and of no significance, neither is a small amount of vaginal blood loss due to an oestrogen withdrawal bleed, nor a milky white vaginal discharge. The labia minora and clitoris may be very prominent in normal pre-term girls.

Abnormalities of the male external genitalia are

much more common. Some mothers (and fathers) are worried by the size of their son's penis, particularly when it is buried in a pad of subpubic fat. The organ is, however, the same size in all races (contrary to popular belief) and is usually 2.5–3.0 cm long. True micropenis is rare, and is often accompanied by other malformations including cryptorchidism. Abnormalities of the shape and extent of the foreskin also spread alarm and despondency; however, so long as the penis is of normal size and the urethral meatus is in the correct place, foreskin morphology is of no clinical relevance.

Hypospadias affects 1:160 newborn, and is usually obvious, since even in minor degrees, the foreskin is abnormally shaped and draws attention to the defect. The urethral orifice can be anywhere on the under surface of the penis right down to the perineum, but in 70 per cent it is in the glans penis or at the corona; if the orifice is proximal to the corona there is usually an associated chordee – a downward curving penis. It is important to check that the urinary stream through the abnormally placed meatus is normal. The management of hypospadias is given on p. 320.

Testicular abnormalities are very common. Many male neonates have a hydrocoele which characteristically is fluctant and transilluminates. No action is required. A hard mass in the scrotum probably means testicular torsion and urgent surgical asessment is required (p. 270). About 3 per cent of males have either one or both testes undescended in the neonatal period. Some are retractile, but if the scrotum on the affected side is hypoplastic, then that testis has never descended. Bilateral undescended testes with a small scrotum should always provoke the examiner to check the infant carefully to ensure that no other stigmata of some dysmorphic syndrome are present.

Herniae are rarely seen in the neonatal period in term babies, but commonly develop during the first month in babies < 1.50 kg birthweight.

SKIN

The skin will have been carefully observed at the start of the examination. Minor abnormalities are common (p. 280 et. seq.), virtually always inconsequential, but a source of anxiety to the mother to whom lesions should always be pointed out and a full explanation given.

TEMPERATURE

If a baby is ill, always remember to take his temperature (this should be a rectal one). Insert the thermometer to about 3 cm but no further. Rectal damage in the neonate from over-enthusiastic insertion of thermometers, or inserting broken thermometers, has been reported. It is, however, exceptionally rare and easily prevented.

THE ROUTINE NEONATAL CLINICAL EXAMINATION (RNCE)

TIMING AND PERSONNEL

All newborn babies should be examined in the neonatal period, ideally in the first 24–48 hours. In the best of all possible worlds this examination should be carried out by someone experienced in neonatal care, not so much because of what he might miss clinically, but because only someone experienced can know how to interpret a finding which is commonly trivial, but might be sinister, and only someone experienced can deal comfortably with the plethora of questions about all aspects of neonatal and paediatric well baby care that the mother is likely to ask.

It is, I believe, very important for those carrying out the examination to have a crystal clear understanding of what they are trying to achieve. They must remember that the patient is asymptomatic, that the midwives will usually have recognised a cleft palate, Down's syndrome, neural tube defects and so on, and that the mother will also have been over her new baby with a fine toothcomb and will already know whether he has all his fingernails, or what colour his eyes are, and whether his external genitalia will pass muster!

There are, therefore, four main functions to the RNCE:

- Detecting serious problems which would otherwise not have been detected, and which merit early assessment and treatment. Basically there are only two common ones, congenital heart disease and congenital dislocation of the hip.
- Checking for droves of very rare but serious conditions, occuring usually in < 1:10 000 live births and which the average paediatrician will find once in a professional lifetime of examining neonates. Examples of these are the enlarged bladder of posterior urethral valves, the posterior abdominal mass of a congenital tumour, a cataract or a dermal sinus leading to the theca.
- Noting, and explaining to the mother, the multitude of normal variations which may be present (Table 7.1).
- Giving the mother a chance to cross-examine the physician about any aspects of the medical care of her baby about which she feels the need for information or reassurance.

It will be clear therefore that the examination must always be done in the presence of the mother.

The physician has to be very careful that he does not over-interpret signs found on the first day in such a way that he subjects the infant to unnecessary investigation and treatment, and the parents to unnecessary anxiety; there is a serious risk that meddlesome interpretation of first-day physical signs can do much more harm than good. In general, therefore, if the examiner finds something on day one which he

TABLE 7.1 Minor abnormalities which may cause maternal alarm

- Skin lesions
    strawberry naevi
    'stork bite'
    milia
    erythema toxicum
    innocent pigmented naevi
    epithelial pearls in the mouth
- Cephalhaematoma
- Subconjunctival haemorrhage
- Peripheral and traumatic cyanosis
- Tongue tie
- Diastasis recti
- Protruberant xiphisternum
- Hydroceles
- Sacral dimple
- Umbilical anomalies, e.g. hernia
- Physiological jaundice
- Snuffles
- Periorbital oedema
- Talipes calcaneo-valgus
- Vaginal skin tag
- Breast enlargement
- Hooded foreskin

thinks is likely to be transient, he should merely keep the infant under observation rather than unjustifiably upsetting the parents with emotive phrases like 'holes-in-the-heart', or 'dislocated-hips' or 'neurologically-a-bit-floppy/stiff'.

If the baby stays in hospital more than 48–72 hours, it is (probably) worth doing a second examination before discharge to check for murmurs and dislocated hips. Thereafter, the baby should have the routine surveillance provided by the GP.

THE EXAMINATION

Ideally the infant should be examined at his mother's

bedside while he is in behavioural state III. The examination should start, as always, by observing the baby's spontaneous behaviour. If that is normal, there is no need to do a further CNS or respiratory examination. Feel the baby all over, looking for lumps and bumps, checking the sutures and fontanelles at the same time. Listen to his heart; in general putting a stethoscope over the lower end of the sternum upsets the baby least and will detect all significant murmurs. Feel the radial and femoral pulses, and palpate the abdomen as described on p. 94. Try to induce the baby to open his mouth and eyes. The former can usually be achieved by gently pressing downwards on his chin, and the latter if he is in stage III is not a problem and in other states can usually be achieved by holding the baby supine and gently rocking his head up and down. Check the genitalia, and turn the baby prone and check his back and natal cleft. Turn him back to supine and examine his hips – leave this until the last since it may make the baby cry, though the object of the exercise is to complete the examination without upsetting him. Finally, measure his OFC. All this can usually be done in 3–4 minutes. The findings should be written in the baby's notes. The routine is the same irrespective of on which day the infant is examined. All that varies is the interpretation of, and action provoked by, positive physical findings.

GESTATIONAL AGE ASSESSMENT

It is my belief that this has become an unnecessarily complex exercise. If a baby is < 1.60 kg, he will be in an NNU and his medical care will be in response to his clinical condition, and assessing his gestation, although of academic and perhaps sociological interest will not influence his management. The same is true for the asymptomatic infant over 2.8–3.0 kg on a PNW. For the 5–10 per cent of babies between these groups it is occasionally of clinical value to assess the gestational age postnatally, in that a small-for-dates 2.00 kg neonate will need to be cared for differently from an appropriate-for-dates pre-term one (Chapter 11). However, in general, even for these babies all that is usually required is an assessment of whether or not the mother's dates are compatible with her infant's appearance, or whether they diverge by the duration of one menstrual cycle. There is little point quibbling about differences in gestational assessment of 7–10 days.

On this basis, I believe that simplicity is of the essence when assessing gestational age, and the following scheme is based on the work of Robinson (1966) and Parkin *et al.* (1976).

NEUROLOGICAL ASSESSMENT

This is best for infants less than 36 weeks (Table 7.2).

Beyond this period one is dependent on cutaneous and soft tissue assessment and the following is that described by Parkin, Hey and Clowes (1976).

TABLE 7.2 Neurological assessment

Reflex	Stimulus	Positive response	Gestation in weeks if reflex is:	
			Absent	Present
Pupil reaction	Light	Pupil constrictions	< 31	29 or more
Glabellar tap	Tap on glabella	Blink	< 34	32 or more
Traction response	Pull up by wrists from supine	Flexion of neck or arm	< 36	33 or more
Neck righting	Rotation of head	Trunk follows	< 37	34 or more

SKIN TEXTURE

Tested by picking up a fold of abdominal skin between finger and thumb and by inspection.

- 0 – very thin with gelatinous feel
- 1 – thin and smooth
- 2 – smooth and of medium thickness; irritation rash and superficial peeling may be present
- 3 – slight thickening and stiff feeling with superficial cracking and peeling especially evident in the hands and feet
- 4 – thick and parchment-like with superficial or deep cracking

SKIN COLOUR

Estimated by inspection when the baby is quiet.
- 0 – dark red
- 1 – uniformly pink
- 2 – pale pink though the colour may vary over different parts of the body: some parts may be very pale
- 3 – pale, nowhere really pink except on the ears, lips, palms and soles

BREAST SIZE

Measured by picking up the breast tissue between finger and thumb.
- 0 – no breast tissue palpable
- 1 – breast tissue palpable on one or both sides, neither being more than 0.5 cm in diameter
- 2 – breast tissue palpable on both sides, one or both being 0.5–1 cm in diameter
- 3 – breast tissue palpable on both sides, one or both being more than 1 cm in diameter

EAR FIRMNESS

Tested by palpation and folding of the upper pinna.
- 0 – pinna feels soft and is easily folded into bizarre positions without springing back into position spontaneously

- 1 – pinna feels soft along the edge and is easily folded but returns slowly to the correct position spontaneously
- 2 – cartilage can be felt to the edge of the pinna though it is thin in places and the pinna springs back after being folded
- 3 – pinna firm with definite cartilage extending peripherally and springs back immediately into position after being folded.

Add up the total scores and the mean gestation for that score is read off Table 7.3.

TABLE 7.3 Assessment of gestational age based on inspection of cutaneous and soft tissue features

Score	Gestational age in weeks
4	34.5
5	36
6	37
7	38.5
8	39.5
9	40
10	41
11–12	41–2

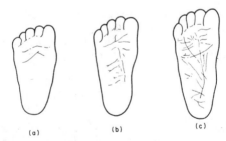

(a)   (b)   (c)

FIGURE 7.4 Diagrammatic representation of sole creases in normal neonates: (a) 36 weeks; (b) 37–38 weeks; (c) 40 weeks (from Gandy, 1992, with permission).

Another feature useful for assessing gestational age is assessing the plantar skin creases in the first hour or two after birth. After this time, all babies tend to get wrinkly as they dry out. In infants of 36 weeks or less there are one or two transverse plantar creases at the level of the metatarsal heads. By 38 weeks these creases have migrated to the mid-point of the sole, and by full term they have reached the heel (Fig. 7.4).

REFERENCES

Clarke, N.M.P. (1994). Role of ultrasound in congenital hip dysplasia. *Archives of Disease in Childhood* **70**, 362–363.

deSwiet M., Peto, J. and Shinebourne, E.A. (1974). Difference between upper and lower limb blood pressure in normal neonates using Doppler technique. *Archives of Disease in Childhood* **49**, 734–736.

Moore, F.H. (1989). Examining infants' hips – can it do harm? *Journal of Bone and Joint Surgery* **71B**, 4–5.

Parkin, J.M., Hey, E.N. and Clowes, J.S. (1976). Rapid assessment of gestational age at birth. *Archives of Disease in Childhood* **51**, 259–263.

Robinson, R.J. (1966). Assessment of gestational age by neurological examination. *Archives of Disease in Childhood* **41**, 437–447.

FURTHER READING

Gandy, G.M. (1992). Examination of the neonate, including gestational age assessment. In: *Textbook of Neonatology*, 2nd Ed. Ed. Roberton, N.R.C. Churchill Livingstone, London and Edinburgh, pp. 199–215.

Roberton, N.R.C. (1984). The routine neonatal clinical examination. In: *Antenatal and Neonatal Screening*. Ed. Wald, N.J. Oxford University Press, pp. 258–282.

8

NEONATAL BIOCHEMICAL SCREENING

Currently all newborn babies in the UK are screened for phenylketonuria and hypothyroidism.

PHENYLKETONURIA

(incidence approximately 1: 10 000)

All babies at 4–7 days of age have a heel prick blood sample analysed for phenylalanine to exclude phenylketonuria. Ideally, the baby should be taking feeds normally. If he is on an inadequate milk intake, he should be retested when his milk intake is normal.

In the Guthrie bacterial inhibition assay, the first test described and still widely used, capillary blood is collected on to an absorbent card (Fig. 8.1). the

TABLE 8.1

Condition	Incidence	Reason for not screening
Histidinaemia	1:17 000	Treatment unnecessary
Homocystinuria	1:150 000	Rare: doubtful if pre-symptomatic treatment is beneficial
Maple syrup urine disease	1:250 000	Rare. Even early dietary treatment leaves most patients severely handicapped
Tyrosinaemia	V.V. rare except in Quebec and Scandinavia	Too rare to be justified

amount of phenylalanine present in one of the blood spots is assayed by its ability to support the growth of *Bacillus subtilis* on an agar plate containing β-thienylalanine which inhibits growth of this organism unless phenylalanine is present. Approximately 1:2000 of all infants are positive on screening. They are recalled, and their plasma phenylalanine remeasured to confirm whether they have classical phenylketonuria or not.

If PKU or a variant is confirmed by a second high phenylalanine level, the baby should be referred to a specialist centre for full investigation and stabilisation on diet.

HYPOTHYROIDISM

(incidence approximately 1:3500)

Using another of the blood spots collected at 6 days on the Guthrie card (Fig. 8.1), a radioimmunoassay is done for thyroid stimulating hormone (TSH) and/or thyroxine (T_4). Most centres have now adopted the primary TSH screening accepting that this will miss cases of secondary hypothyroidism. Those with a high TSH are recalled for further testing. This is required in 0.2–0.3 per cent of infants tested.

The incidence of hypothyroidism detected in this way is about double that previously identified clinically in early infancy, presumably due to the fact that some neonates, particularly if pre-term, have transient hypothyroidism, whereas others have only marginally subnormal thyroid function which would not otherwise have presented till later in childhood.

All infants confirmed as hypothyroid should be treated and carefully followed up.

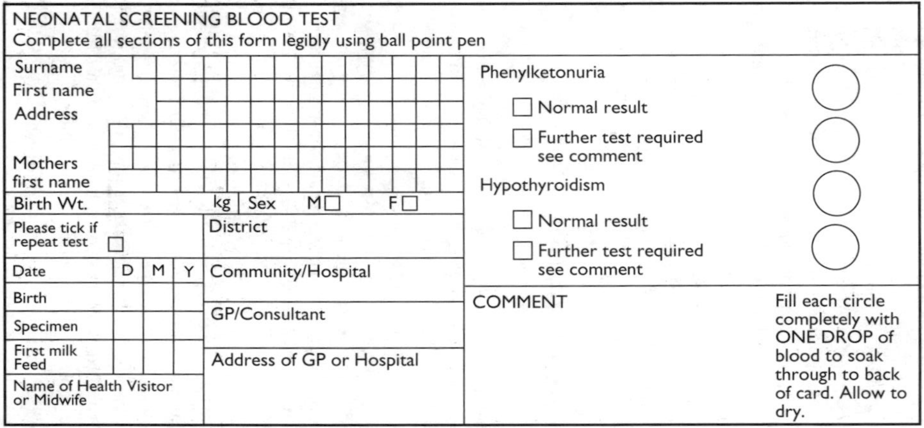

NEONATAL SCREENING BLOOD TEST
Complete all sections of this form legibly using ball point pen

Surname
First name
Address
Mothers first name
Birth Wt. kg | Sex M ☐ F ☐
Please tick if repeat test ☐
District

Date	D	M	Y
Birth			
Specimen			
First milk Feed			

Community/Hospital
GP/Consultant
Address of GP or Hospital
Name of Health Visitor or Midwife

Phenylketonuria
☐ Normal result
☐ Further test required see comment

Hypothyroidism
☐ Normal result
☐ Further test required see comment

COMMENT

Fill each circle completely with ONE DROP of blood to soak through to back of card. Allow to dry.

FIGURE 8.1 Card currently used for collection of blood for Guthrie test.

OTHER INBORN ERRORS OF AMINO ACID METABOLISM

In some parts of the UK and overseas, maple syrup urine disease, homocystinuria, histidinaemia and tyrosinaemia are screened for, either by modifications of the Guthrie bacterial inhibition type of assay or by plasma chromatography or fluorimetry.

However, these conditions (Table 8.1) are all rare, difficult to treat or, in the case of histidinaemia, of doubtful clinical significance. It is questionable therefore, whether the addition of extra screening tests for these conditions is cost effective.

GALACTOSAEMIA

(incidence 1:40–60 000)

Infants with this condition may become ill in the neonatal period before the time of screening. However, the test for galactose 1-phosphate uridyl transferase deficiency is easily and cheaply carried out on red cells from a Guthrie card, or any other blood specimens. Despite the comparative rarity of galactosaemia, it is probably worthwhile screening routinely, though this is not yet routine in many parts of Britain.

CYSTIC FIBROSIS

(incidence 1:2000)

This is the most common lethal inherited disease in Caucasians. Whether ot nor neonatal screening is justified hinges largely on whether there are benefits from detecting and treating this condition in its pre-symtomatic stage. Much of the evidence supports this view, but screening is as yet not universal in Britain. Blood spots obtained from the Guthrie test (Fig. 8.1) can be analysed for immunoreactive trypsin (IRT) which is markedly raised in most neonates with cystic fibrosis. Preliminary studies suggest that the test is very specific with a recall rate of only 0.5 per cent and very few false positive or false negative results.

OTHER CONDITIONS

Screening using the Guthrie card is also available for Duchenne muscular dystrophy (using creatine kinase) and congenital adrenal hyperplasia (using 17–hydroxy progesterone). In Japan, 6-month-olds are screened for neuroblastoma by assay of VMA in urine. None of these procedures has become routine except in high-incidence areas.

CLINICAL SCREENING

The routine neonatal clinical examination as a screening test is described on p. 106. Screening for congenital dislocation of the hip using ultrasound is discussed on p. 105, and hearing testing on p. 100.

9

INFANT FEEDING

LACTATION

(Glasier and McNeilly, 1990)

A characteristic feature of the class Mammalia, as their name implies, is the possession of breasts, vestigial in the male, but developed in the female to produce a milk uniquely suited in volume and composition for feeding her baby.

During pregnancy the glandular tissue and ducts within the breasts enlarge. These are stimulated by the rise in oestrogens, progesterone, gonadotrophins and human placental lactogen, thereby priming the organ for lactation postnatally. Prolactin also rises steadily during pregnancy, but its action to stimulate milk production is inhibited by progesterone. Small amounts of fluid are produced in the breast throughout the latter part of gestation, and some leaks from the breast at this stage. However, more of it is released from the breast in the first 48–72 hours postpartum before lactogenesis (milk production) occurs. This early fluid is the colostrum.

Immediately after delivery, the sudden fall in the levels of progesterone, as well as oestrogen and human placental lactogen, coupled with a further rise in prolactin production results in the secretion of milk in to the aveoli of the breast. This is called lactogenesis. Continued production of prolactin is, thereafter, dependent on continuing suckling, and nipple stimulation is one of the two powerful stimuli to prolactin production.

The other important stimulus to successful milk

production is ensuring that the breast is emptied at each feed, since the retention of milk in the alveoli would appear to reduce milk production probably by inhibiting fatty acid synthesis within the breast. The effect of frequent suckling on prolactin production, and the need to empty the breast at each feed, clearly have important implications for the management of breast-feeding in the immediate postpartum period (see below).

Milk which has been secreted into the breast alveoli is actively expelled, the so-called let down reflex, into the ducts of the breast and then out of the nipple by active contraction of the myoepithelial cells which surround all these structures. Contraction of these cells is stimulated by oxytocin released by the maternal pituitary both in response to suckling and to auditory or visual stimuli from her baby, such as a cry of just the sight of him looking hungry. Suckling also physically squeezes milk out of the lactiferous ducts under the areola, and also removes some milk from the breast simply by suction. However, it is important to remember that the let down reflex does actually expel milk into the baby's mouth which is often of major benefit to those neonates with, for example, a harelip and cleft palate who have difficulties sucking.

Careful studies of women with established lactation have shown that primarily under the influence of the let down reflex most milk is expelled from the breast in the first 4–6 minutes of a feed. Suckling beyond that time, while it may have a role in promoting prolactin and oxytocin secretion, is more for the mutual emotional gratification of the mother and baby.

The physiological changes which result in adequate milk production take time to get underway after birth, with the result that for the first 48–72 hours very little fluid is produced by the breast; however, the colostrum which is produced, is of great value to the neonate since it is very rich in hormones, white blood cells, minerals and particularly in immunoglobulins. Colostral immunoglobulins, and the lower concentration (but greater volume) of immunoglobulins which are present in mature breast milk, help to protect the neonate against infection (see p. 124).

After about 48 hours postpartum, the milk 'comes in' to the mother's breast, a fact which she is often acutely aware of as her breasts become full, sometimes painfully full and engorged. From that time onwards, so long as the baby sucks regularly, stimulating prolactin production, and the breasts are regularly emptied, the mother can go on producing milk for years if necessary.

The physiological changes outlined above which result in milk production can occur after delivery at any gestation, even after miscarriages at 14–16 weeks gestation, though the amount of breast engorgement or milk produced is usually very small before 24–26 weeks of gestation. Lactation can even be created artificially in women who have not been pregnant but have adopted a neonate whom they wish to breastfeed. This is done with oestrogen priming, coupled with the use of drugs which stimulate prolactin production (e.g. thyrotrophin releasing hormone [TRH], or metoclopramide) followed by regular suckling. Such 'relactation' is more easy to achieve if the mother has lactated in the past.

BREAST MILK COMPOSITION

(Table 9.1)

There is no such thing as standard breast milk. The composition of the milk varies with the gestation at delivery, the postnatal age, the mother's diet, from day-to-day in an individual woman, and in between the start and the end of a feed. In general, the shorter the gestation, the higher the concentration of protein, calories and sodium, and the longer lactation has been going on after delivery at any gestation, the

TABLE 9.1 Milk composition: cows' v breast milk

	Cow	Mature breast milk*
Carbohydrate (lactose) (g/100 ml)	4.6	7.0–7.4
Fat (g/100 ml)	3.9	3.8–4.2
Protein (g/100 ml)	3.4	1.1–1.45
(Casein:lactalbumin ratio)	4:1	2:3
Calories/100 ml	67	68–70
Na$^+$ (mmol/l)	23	6.4
K$^+$ (mmol/l)	40	15
Ca^{++} (mg%)	124	35
PO$_4$ (mg%)	98	15
Fe^{++} (mg%)	0.05	0.08
Vit A (μg/100 ml)	17–38	60
Vit D (μg/100 ml)	0.02	0.01
Vit E (μg/100 ml)	90	350
Folic acid (μg/100 ml)	3.7	5.2

*Data from several sources.

lower the concentration of protein and sodium, though calories are well sustained by a rising fat and carbohydrate content. Thus, the first-week milk of a mother delivering at 30 weeks is more concentrated than that of a woman delivering at 40 weeks. Five months later, they will be producing a milk – the so-called mature milk – which will be virtually identical in both women.

Milk collected at the start of a feed, the fore milk, has a lower fat, and therefore correspondingly lower calorie content than that produced at the end of the feed, the hind milk.

NUTRIENT CONTENT

Lactose is the only carbohydrate present in human milk, and its concentration varies very little from woman to woman. The protein is predominantly α-lactalbumin with much smaller amounts of casein (which is the predominant protein in cows' milk).

Included in the total protein are anti-infection agents such as immunoglobulins and lactoferrin (see below). In addition, there are free amino acids in breast milk, which together with urea, creatinine, uric acid and some ammonia form about 35 per cent of its total nitrogen content.

The fat content of breast milk is shown in Table 9.1. In general, the triglycerides in breast milk fat contain more unsaturated fatty acids than cows' milk. This is, however, variable and depends on the maternal diet. Women who eat a lot of polyunsaturated fat produce milk with a lot of polyunsaturated fats in it, whereas those taking a lot of animal fat will have a more saturated fat in their EBM. The mineral and vitamin composition of breast milk is given in Table 9.1. It should be noted that the levels of iron and vitamin D are particularly low.

The fetus is, however, an effective parasite on the maternal iron stores (p. 23), and at term, irrespective of maternal race and iron status, will have enough iron in his tissues, together with the small iron intake from exclusive breast-feeding, to last for the first 6 months of his life. Thereafter, iron intake in exclusively breast-fed infants is inadequate, and any infants still exclusively breast-fed beyond 6 months should reveive iron supplements. If the mother is vitamin D deficient, then the neonate will also be deficient and may develop neonatal hypocalcaemia. This can, however, be prevented by vitamin D supplementation in at-risk pregnant women. If the infant of a woman likely to be at risk from vitamin D deficiency is going to be exclusively breast-fed for more than a few weeks, he should receive vitamin D supplements postnatally particularly if, because of racial pigmentation or social factors, such as clothing and the time he spends outside exposed to sunlight, he is unlikely to be able to synthesise vitamin D in his skin – the mechanism by which most Caucasian infants avoid rickets if they are exclusively breast-fed beyond 4–6 months of age.

ANTI-INFECTIVE AGENTS

Breast milk contains a multitude of anti-infective agents (Table 9.2). The predominant immunoglobulin is IgA; whether the IgG has any function remains speculative. There is an entero-mammary circulation of B lymphocytes in the mother, so that lymphocytes stimulated in her bowel by enteric pathogens rapidly migrate to her breast and release their secretory IgA into her milk. The concentration of anti-infectious agents, in particular IgA, is highest in colostrum (approx. $2\,g/litre$) and then falls off rapidly in the first week to levels around $0.8\,g/litre$ in mature milk. However, as milk production increases the infant still ingests considerable quantities of IgA.

TABLE 9.2 Anti-infection factors in breast milk

- Immunoglobulins (IgA, IgG)
- Complement
- Lysozyme
- Lactoferrin
- Vitamin B_{12} and folate binding proteins
- Antistaphylococcal factor
- Protease inhibitors (protecting IgA)
- Bifidus factor (encouraging lactobacillus growth)
- Interferon
- Antiviral factors
- WBC

Lactoferrin is a powerful iron binding protein which, by chelating all the iron in the gut lumen, denies it to the enteric bacterial flora which requires iron for proliferation. In addition to non-specific anti-infectious agents such as complement, lysozyme and interferon, an important anti-infectious property of breast milk is its low protein content. This makes it a poor buffer, and the stools of breast-fed infants are more acidic than those of bottle-fed ones. An acid pH in colonic contents inhibits the multiplication of enteric organisms. The modern low-protein formulae have this beneficial effect to some extent.

Breast milk also contains factors (e.g. the bifidus factor) which encourage the growth of non-pathogenic organisms (e.g. lactobacilli), in the gut lumen, rather than pathogenic ones (e.g. *E. coli*, p. 84).

Another important anti-infection feature of EBM is its cleanliness. It is, however *not* sterile since it usually contains the normal skin commensals from the mother's breast which may be in the ducts of her breast just below the nipple and areola, and are certainly on her areola when the baby takes it into his mouth. Nevertheless, this is very much cleaner than bottle milk prepared in unhygienic conditions, but probably offers few advantages in the modern sanitised home.

OTHER FACTORS

Breast milk contains desirable substances such as hormones, biological amines, growth factors and enzymes, as well as less desirable substances like drugs and environmental toxins (such as the by-products of cigarette smoking) ingested by the mother. The effect of many of these agents is speculative, but some drugs should undoubtedly be avoided (p. 41 et. seq.).

VOLUME

Once lactation is fully established, studies from many parts of the world on mothers of very different socio-economic, ethnic and cultural backgrounds have shown a very consistent average milk production of 750–800 ml/day with a range of 500–1200 ml. In the earlier weeks of lactation with a 3–4 kg baby needing 150–170 ml/kg/24 hours, the supply is tailored to demand in response to the physiological stimuli of suckling and breast emptying, but once the ceiling of production at, say, 800 ml/24 hours has been reached, this cannot be increased by the techniques used to stimulate failing lactation in the first few days or weeks (p. 156).

COWS' MILK AND COWS' MILK BASED FORMULAE

Cows' milk in its unaltered form (Table 9.1) is totally inappropriate as a food for the human infant < 6 months of age and probably inappropriate for those 6–12 months old (American Academy of Pediatrics, 1992). Until the mid-1970s most of the cows' milk derived formulae were only marginally altered from what was produced by the cow, other than by adding lactose, sometimes iron and vitamin D, and often some chemical agent to help in the physical preparation of the powder and its reconstitution into liquid milk. There were three main problems with these old formulae, and with unadulterated cows' milk:

- They had an inappropriately high protein, and in particular casein, content causing hyperosmolarity, acidaemia and a raised blood urea.
- They had an inappropriately high sodium content, resulting in hypernatraemia, particularly if the infant became even mildly dehydrated.
- They had an inappropriately high phosphate content, causing hyperphosphataemia in the neonate, followed by hypocalcaemia and convulsions.

These problems were exacerbated if the mothers made up the milk in to concentrated a form from the powder – the 'one for the pot' mentality.

Since the mid-1970s, however, the manufacturers have enormously improved their products in many ways including:

- reducing the total protein content;
- increasing the lactalbumin to casein ratio (whey: curds) of the protein to that found in breast milk
- reducing the sodium and phosphate content;
- increasing the iron and vitamin D content;

- improving the fatty acid composition to something like that of breast milk.

As a result, the metabolic complications listed above are no longer seen in bottle-fed babies, though will of course occur if the neonate is fed on unadultered cows' milk or 'doorstep' milk as delivered by the dairyman.

None of the formulae (Table 9.3) contain hormones, amines, amino acids, or anti-infectious agents (though their low protein content does encourage colonic acidity, p. 125). Nor do they contain drugs, nicotine or alcohol, but they may contain environmental toxins ingested by the cow and not removed by the milk processing procedure.

Many of these milks come in two forms: a powdered milk for reconstitution with boiled water (not boiling), and a 'ready-to-feed' (RTF) liquid preparation made up in 100 ml bottles. There are marginal differences between the composition of the RTF preparations and the reconstituted powdered milks, but these are of no practical or clinical importance.

TABLE 9.3 Composition of commonly used whey-based milks

	SMA Gold Cap	Cow & Gate Premium*	Farley's Osterfeed	Milupa Aptamil
Carbohydrate (g/100 ml)	7.2	7.5(6.9)	7.0	7.3
Fat (g/100 ml)	3.6	3.6(3.5)	3.82	3.6
Protein (g/100 ml)	1.5	1.4(1.8)	1.45	1.5
(Casein:lactalbumin ratio)	2:3	2:3	2:3	2:3
Calories/100 ml	67	66	68	67
Na^+ (mmol/litre)	7.0	7.8(9.6)	8.5	7.8
K^+ (mmol/litre)	16.6	16.6	14.5	21.7
Ca^{++} (mg%)	46	54(48)	35	59
PO_4^{111} (mg%)	33	27	29	35
Fe^{++} (mg%)	0.8	0.5	0.65	0.7
Vitamin A (μg/100 ml)	75	80	100	61
Vitamin D (μg/100 ml)	1.1	1.1	1.0	1.0
Vitamin E (μg/100 ml)	740	1100	480	700
Folic acid (μg/100 ml)	8.0	10	3.4	10.0

*Figures in brackets show the composition of ready-to-feed preparations.

These whey-based milks should be used in babies over 1.80 kg for whom breast-feeding is not possible. As can be seen (Table 9.3), there are only tiny variations in the composition of the various products. Although the sales patter of the manufacturers' salesmen may try to convince you that these differences are of clinical or nutritional significance, this is not the case. All the milks are to all intents and purposes the same. There is, therefore, no point whatsoever in swapping babies with various feeding problems from one formula to another.

PRE-TERM FOLLOW-ON FORMULAE

Studies have shown that the ex-prem once discharged home drinks very large quantities of milk – up to 300 ml/kg/24 hours, and commonly exceeds 220–230 ml/kg/24 hours. In this way, they achieve some catch-up growth. One approach to handling this problem is to produce special post-discharge formulae for pre-term babies, and two of these are now available (Table 9.4). Their use should be limited to babies less than 2.00 kg birthweight, but can be used for them until they are 9 months old.

TABLE 9.4 Composition of pre-term follow-on milks

	Premcare (Farley's)	Nutriprem II (Cow & Gate)
Carbohydrate (g/100 ml)	7.3	7.5
Fat (g/100 ml)	4.0	4.1
Protein (g/100 ml)	1.85	1.80
Calories/100 ml	72	74
Na^+ (mmol/l)	9.6	10.4
K^+ (mmol/l)	20	18.7
Ca^{++} (mg%)	70	80
$PO_4^{\,III}$ (mg%)	35	40
Fe^{++} (mg%)	650	1100
Vitamin A (μg/100 ml)	100	107
Vitamin D (μg/100 ml)	1.3	1.6
Vitamin E (μg/100 ml)	1.5	1.2
Folic acid (μg/100 ml)	25	20

CURD-BASED AND FOLLOW-ON FORMULAE

All the four major UK milk-producing companies now produce two other types of infant formula – their curd-based milks for early infancy, but outside the neonatal period, and their follow-on formulae for babies over 6 months, for whom it is now generally agreed that 'doorstep' milk is inappropriate until they are over 1 year old. The curd-based preparations (Table 9.5) have slightly higher concentrations of almost everything and are said to 'satisfy' apparently hungry crying babies of 4–6 weeks or more who, while fed whey-based milks, are fractious after feeds appear to be still hungry, or are not gaining weight adequately.

TABLE 9.5 Composition of commonly used curd-based milks

	SMA White	Cow & Gate Nutrilon Plus	Farley's Ostermilk 2	Milupa Milumil
Carbohydrate (g/100 ml)	7.0	7.2	8.6*	8.4†
Fat (g/100 ml)	3.6	3.4	2.6	3.1
Protein (g/100 ml)	1.6	1.7	1.7	1.9
Casein:lactalbumin ratio	4:1	4:1	4:1	4:1
Calories/100 ml	67	66	65	69
Na^+ (mmol/l)	9.6	10.9	10.9	10.4
K^+ (mmol/l)	20.4	23	22	21.7
Ca^{++} (mg%)	56	80	61	71
PO_4^{III} (mg%)	44	47	49	55
Fe^{++} (mg%)	0.8	0.5	0.65	0.43
Vitamin A (μg/100 ml)	75	80	97	57
Vitamin D (μg/100 ml)	1.1	1.1	1.0	1.0
Vitamin E (μg/100 ml)	740	1100	460	800
Folic acid (μg/100 ml)	8.0	10.0	3.2	5.0

*5–8 g of carbohydrate is maltodextrin, a glucose polymer.
†1.3 g of carbohydrate is maltodextrin and 1.1 g is amylose.

The follow-on formulae should not be used until babies are 6 months old or more, and these have still higher contents of protein and minerals (Table 9.6), which clearly precludes their use in younger babies –

TABLE 9.6 Composition of follow-on milks for babies over 6 months

	SMA Progress	Cow & Gate Junior Milk	Boots/Farley's Milk drink	Milupa Step-up
Carbohydrate (g/100 ml)	7.8	8.0	6.43	7.2
Fat (g/100 ml)	3.0	3.0	3.41	3.8
Protein (g/100 ml)	2.2	2.0	2.15	1.8
Calories/100 ml	67	67	65	70
Na$^+$ (mmol/l)	14.4	13.1	12.7	10
K$^+$ (mmol/l)	27.4	25.6	24.8	22
Ca^{++} (mg%)	90	72	69	88
PO$_4^{|||}$ (mg%)	62	59	58	50
Fe^{++} (mg%)	1.3	0.7	0.85	1.3
Vitamin A (mg/100 ml)	75	80	130	60
Vitamin D (mg/100 ml)	1.2	1.1	1.3	2.1
Vitamin E (mg/100 ml)	740	480	550	1100
Folic (μg/100 ml)	8.0	7.0	3.9	11.0

and they are in a sense, therefore, outside the scope of this book.

It is of course of crucial importance that the powdered milks are always reconstituted in the correct way, and that the manufacturers' instructions on the packets are followed exactly, otherwise the milk fed to the baby will not have the acceptable composition listed in Tables 9.3–9.6. There are obvious dangers both in making the milk too concentrated (complications as for the older formulae or 'doorstep milk') or making it too dilute (malnutrition, vitamin and electrolyte deficiencies).

SOYA MILKS

These milks are based on a protein derived from the soya bean. Appropriate lipid, carbohydrate, mineral and vitamin supplements are then added (Table 9.7). Some doubts remain about the nutritional adequacy of the protein preparations, though deficiency conditions such as hypochloraemic alkalosis which occurred in the past have been avoided by appropriate modifications to the formulae. I am totally unimpressed by the data suggesting that using soya milk as an alternative to cows' milk based formulae in the neonatal period has any value in reducing the subsequent incidence of atopic disease in the baby, and it has to be remembered that allergy to soya protein can be just as much a hazard as allergy to cows' milk. I do not believe, therefore, that soya milks have any routine role in neonatal nutrition.

TABLE 9.7 Composition of special milks

	Cow & Gate Nutrilon Soya	SMA Wysoy	Farley's Ostersoy	Goat
Protein (g%)	1.8	1.8	1.95	3.5
Fat (g%)	3.6	3.6	3.8	4.65
Carbohydrate (g%)	7.1	6.9	7.0	4.7
Calories/100 ml	66	67	70	67
Na^+ (mmol/l)	7.8	8.3	10.9	14
K^+ (mmol/l)	17	18.4	19.2	46
Ca^{++} (mg%)	54	67	56	128
PO_4^{III} (mg%)	27	50	37	104.5
Fe^{++} (mg%)	0.81	0.8	0.65	0.5
Vitamin A (μg/100 ml)	80	75	100	71
Vitamin D (μg%)	1.1	1.1	1.1	0.06
Folic acid (μg/100 ml)	10	8.0	3.5	0.6

OTHER MILKS

The trendy, macrobiotic diet, vegetarian segment of the population occasionally show a predilection for foisting goats' milk on their offspring. This product (Table 9.7) is not only highly unlikely to be microbiologically safe – the animals are not regularly brucellin or TB tested, and the production methods are less likely to be as sanitised as those used by the infant milk manufacturing industry – but furthermore, it is

nutritionally extremely dangerous with a high osmo-
lar load, worse in fact than unadulterated cows' milk,
an adverse electrolyte composition and virtually no
folic acid. It is highly allergenic. *This form of child abuse
must be prevented.* Milks used in other parts of the
world from animals such as the camel, sheep or yak
are equally unsatisfactory.

THE BREAST VERSUS BOTTLE CONTROVERSY

This is a matter of great medical, scientific and social
interest, and the pros and cons will be discussed
below. What is being compared is breast-feeding with
the use of one of the newer cows' milk based formulae designed for full term neonates (Table 9.3),
since soya milk and unaltered cows', goats', seals',
camels' or gorillas' milks are totally inappropriate for
the human neonate.

ALLERGY

Ten to 20 per cent of the adult population suffers
from or have suffered from some form of
allergic/atopic disease such as asthma, eczema, food
allergy, hay fever or allergic skin eruptions. The tendency to develop allergic disease is inherited, and
whether or not symptoms develop is likely to depend
on environmental factors. The literature on whether
breast-feeding or bottle-feeding is one of these environmental factors is controversial and confusing.
That up to 1988 is well reviewed by Kramer (1988)
and nothing published since has clarified the issue.
One of the main problems in studying the topic is
the ubiquitous nature of environmental allergens
which may affect the baby from the time of birth irrespective of feeding practice, and the fact that dietary
allergens ingested by the pregnant woman such as
cows' milk and eggs may cross the placenta, and once

she starts to lactate they enter her milk.

The following conclusions may, however, be reached from the literature.

- In the family without a previous history of allergic disease breast-feeding does not significantly reduce the incidence of subsequent allergic disease including asthma in the new baby.
- In atopic families exclusive breast-feeding appears to offer little if any protection unless other environmental and dietary allergens are also avoided by mother and baby in the first 6 months, and then it only protects against eczema.
- Some studies even suggest a higher incidence of allergic disease following prolonged breast-feeding (Savilahti *et al.*, 1987).
- If an atopic woman really wants to have an impact on atopic disease in her baby she should take a hypoallergenic diet for the last half of pregnancy and while breast-feeding.
- The specific entity of primary cows' milk protein intolerance – as opposed to that which develops secondary to gastroenteritis – can be largely avoided by early breast-feeding.

ANTI-INFECTIOUS PROPERTIES

This has always been the prime reason for recommending breast-feeding and in the developing world, bottle-feeding is the next best thing to a death sentence from infection, though it may be that this relates simply to the cleanliness of breast milk and the impossibility of sustaining the adequate standards of hygiene required for bottle milk preparation if you are illiterate, and live in a cardboard hut without mains water, drainage or electricity!

However in the socio-economically privileged Western world with piped water, mains drainage, refrigerators and virtually 100 per cent literacy it is difficult to find good evidence, while allowing for other socio-economic correlates of bottle-feeding known to increase the risk of infection like social class, over-crowding, poor nutrition and maternal smoking. If there is an anti-infection benefit from breast milk in the UK it is probably minor, and limited to enteric infections and perhaps otitis media.

CONTRACEPTION

Breast-feeding is not a complete contraceptive. However, women fully breast-feeding for the first 6 months who remain amenorrhoeic are very unlikely (1.7 per cent) to become pregnant (Short *et al.*, 1991). Other breast-feeding women wishing to ensure that they do not become pregnant should use contraceptives either of a barrier form or the progesterone only mini pill. Taking an oestrogen containing contraceptive will not harm the baby, but is likely to reduce the daily milk production by 100–150 ml.

CONVENIENCE, COST, SOCIAL AND PSYCHOLOGICAL FACTORS

Whether a woman finds it more convenient to breast-feed or not is an intensely personal matter. For some women, always having a supply of warm milk with her greatly outweighs any embarrassment about feeding in public, or the risk of a damp dress front. Fortunately, there is now an infinitely more liberal and rational approach to providing mothers with facilities to breast-feed at work and in public than was the case 10–15 years ago. Nevertheless, breast-feeding still falls off more rapidly in women who return to full-time employment than in those who stay at home.

Breast-feeding almost inevitably means more feeds per day, and this is socially more tying. However, breast milk can be expressed in to a bottle and given by the father or other caretakers if necessary. In the first 1–2 weeks of life, a breast-fed infant tends to settle into a pattern of 7–8 feeds per day whereas bottle-fed babies require only 5–6. One additional manifestation of this increased frequency of feeds is that night-time feeds are needed for longer in breast-fed infants.

Breast-feeding is probably cheaper than bottle-feeding. To sustain lactation a woman probably needs 300–500 calories' worth of food per day. This can be of cheap foods, e.g. 100 g of carbohydrate as bread or potato and a little protein costing, say, 20–25 pence, whereas to give 600 ml of one of the standard powdered milks (150 ml/kg/24 hours) to a 4 kg baby will cost 2–3 times more.

Breast-feeding is probably better for the mother's figure; some of the fat laid down during pregnancy is, arguing teleologically, a calorie reserve to sustain breast-feeding postnatally. Losing this weight is more likely to occur if the mother breast-feeds, than if she does not.

It is clearly nonsense to suggest that a bottle-fed baby feels unloved, or that the lack of intimate mother–baby contact implicit in breast-feeding has any long-term deleterious emotional effect on the child. It is difficult to see how a bottle-fed baby cuddled to his mother during a feed, hearing her heart beat and voice can feel anything other than loved. In these days of sexual equality, the emotional needs of the father who wishes to be involved in infant care but is denied the satisfaction of breast-feeding his baby can only be assuaged by the mother expressing milk in to a bottle; whether this is justified is a matter of intrafamilial negotiation.

There are also quite definite emotional and psychological disadvantages to breast-feeding, and it will not be lost on the observant reader of pages 151–165, that the vast majority of the feeding problems and traumas in the first weeks occur exclusively in breast-fed babies. Engorged breasts, cracked nipples, hungry screaming babies who won't fix at the nipple or suck are the almost exclusive preserve of the demoralised tired and tearful breast-feeding mother. By and large, if you stick a rubber teat in a baby's mouth, he slurps down his formula, burps and goes off in to a blissful sleep – as does his mother. Nevertheless, for many women, it is clear that the emotional delight they feel when feeding their baby at their breast is one of the most intensely rewarding and satisfying activities they ever experience, and they should be encouraged to enjoy this. For other women, the chomping of a powerful set of 4 kg jaws on a tender cracked nipple evokes different emotions.

COT DEATH

The data relating bottle milk to cot death is also far from impressive because of the usual difficulties in teasing out the socio-economic correlates which are common to both bottle-feeding and cot death. Exclusively breast-fed babies can certainly be cot deaths, and there is probably no protective effect from breast-feeding *per se* (HMSO, 1993). Furthermore, the risk of cot death should never be used to badger a woman into breast-feeding her baby.

DRUGS AND TOXINS

Environmental toxins get in to both breast milk and cows' milk, though it is doubtful if these are of any importance. The danger of drugs in breast milk is overstated and is dealt with in detail on p. 41 et. seq.

FAILURE TO THRIVE

(see also poor weight gain, p. 162)

All paediatricians see a steady sprinkling, often of social class 1, well-educated women with marasmic, 2–3 month old, breast-fed infants, who clearly have just not been taking enough milk, and yet have not voiced their starvation by regularly howling for food.

Such babies gobble down complementary bottle-feeds and promptly thrive. These complementary bottle-feeds can be continued if the mother is an obsessive breast-feeder, but in most cases it is usually sensible to swap over to all formula feeds, unless the routines outlined on p. 156 result in an increase in milk production and a marked weight gain in the baby.

Those caring for the exclusively breast-fed baby after discharge from a maternity hospital have, therefore, a major responsibility to ensure that he is gaining weight consistently at 200 g/week (approx. 30 g/24 hours, p. 83).

INTELLIGENCE

There are no studies on term babies that compare intellectual outcome of breast- or bottle-fed babies which provide acceptable controls for the beneficial socio-economic variables likely to accrue in breast-fed neonates. However, ill term babies fed by tube with EBM may have a better IQ on follow-up than those fed on formula.

MATERNAL ILLNESS

The interaction of lactation and various chronic maternal illnesses is described in Chapter 3, as are problems of breast-feeding in the presence of acute maternal perinatal illness and infection. If a mother is acutely ill, it is obviously much easier for the father or other family members to take over the responsibility for bottle-feeding. If the illness is likely to be short-lived, the mother can sustain her lactation by expressing milk which can then be given by bottle. However, any acute maternal illness is likely to reduce her milk production because of poor prolactin production combined with stress, often coupled with a poor maternal fluid and caloric intake. If her illness is prolonged, the continuation of lactation is adversely affecting the maternal condition, or if the baby who has stayed on the breast is failing to thrive, lactation should be abandoned and bottle-feeding commenced.

NUTRITIONAL COMPARISONS

There is no evidence that term infants fed on the modern formulae are in any way nutritionally disadvantaged. There is no evidence that the absence of hormones or free amino acids in the artificial milk matters, nor that the different fat content has any implications in the short term, or for degenerative arterial disease in the long term. In the developing world and in Western communities, exclusively bottle-fed babies are bigger than exclusively breast-fed ones (Dewey *et al.*, 1992). Whether this has any long-term implications or benefits is unknown. Breast milk is undoubtedly deficient in vitamin D and iron; there is no evidence that this causes problems in the first 6 months for the exclusively breast-fed Caucasian infant of a well-nourished mother in northern latitudes; however, this may not be the case in the infant of an African or Indian mother whose vitamin D status is less secure.

WEIGHT LOSS, JAUNDICE, HYPOGLYCAEMIA

It is now clear that breast-fed babies, probably for multiple reasons, lose more weight in the neonatal period than bottle-fed babies, and become more jaundiced. Neither of these clinical entities should cause problems, since the extra weight loss is of no significance, and is virtually always within the allowed 10 per cent (p. 83). The jaundice rarely reaches levels at which a rational paediatrician instigates dietary changes or phototherapy (p. 242). Prolonged jaundice may also be seen in breast-fed infants and is described fully in Chapter 17. The diagnosis can be proved by noting that the jaundice clears when breast-feeding is stopped for 24–48 hours, but this is rarely if ever justified.

Hypoglycaemia is a major risk in the first 24–48 hours in breast-fed, small-for-dates babies and infants of diabetic mothers in whom special precautions are justified (pp. 184, 210). It can also occur very rarely if breast-feeding is going really badly in a well-grown full term infant (pp. 165 and 278) and always requires treatment.

All these problems with a baby may also cause maternal anxiety despite reassurance, and this may be heightened if ill-advised interference or therapy is prescribed. Anxiety reduces prolactin and milk secretion, and a vicious circle of low milk production, hypoglycaemia, jaundice, maternal anxiety and even lower milk production is therefore easily created.

SUMMARY

If we take an overview of all these factors discussed above it is clear that in the developing world breast-feeding is essential to prevent a horrendous infant mortality from infectious disease. In the developed world, however, where the role of breast-feeding in preventing infection is much less clear the arguments for and against breast-feeding add up as follows.

The advantages of breast feeding are:
- a reduction in the incidence of cows' milk protein intolerance;
- a slight reduction in gastroenteritis and perhaps otitis media;
- cheaper;
- better for the mother's figure;
- better for the mother's psyche so long as everything goes well; potentially devastating otherwise.

The disadvantages are:
- more socially tying, and more feeds needed, including more night feeds;
- transmission of drugs;

- lack of paternal involvement;
- poor contraception;
- small risk of failure to thrive, hypoglycaemia, and perhaps iron and vitamin D deficiency;
- increased risk of jaundice; not medically important, but anxiety provoking;
- poorer weight gain in infancy.

Looking at it this way, the benefits of breast-feeding are much less clear-cut particularly from the baby's point of view, and this should certainly be borne in mine when counselling a woman who wishes to bottle-feed her baby. We have no hard facts to pressurise her in to changing her mind.

However, the argument does go that breast milk is designed for human babies, and where term babies are concerned this cannot be argued against. For the woman who watches her baby's weight, is not on drugs and is not disconcerted by the social ties imposed by breast-feeding, breast-feeding certainly does the baby no major harm, it may protect him from some infections and it will probably save the family money, improve the mother's figure, and give her an intense feeling of personal gratification. These last three factors are true of precious little else in Britain in 1996! Like most paediatricians, therefore, I am very pro-breast-feeding.

THE PRACTICALITIES OF FEEDING NEONATES

BOTTLE-FEEDING

Which milk?

The baby should be given one of the standard infant formulae (see Table 9.3), usually the one provided on contract to the hospital. In general if the mother has a fixation on one of the other milks her whims should be indulged, though there is no significant difference between any of the products listed in Table 9.3. For ex-prem babies the special formulae designed for their use (Table 9.4) should be used.

Starting feeds

If a mother has elected to bottle-feed her baby, this should be started once a baby reaches the postnatal ward (PNW) or if the baby is at home once he wakes up and appears hungry. In most PNWs there is usually some scheduled time at which bottle-feeds are offered, usually on a 4-hourly basis. Although, as will be outlined below when discussing breast-feeding, there is no biological justification for the 4-hourly schedule, bottle-fed babies commonly settle in to such a pattern. The newly delivered baby destined for bottle-feeds should, therefore, be offered a bottle at the first scheduled feeding time after his admission to the PNW. If he is fast asleep, there is no need to do anything. If he is at home, wait 2–4 hours until he wakes. Remember that breast-fed babies receive few calories for the first 24–48 hours until the mother's milk 'comes in', and that the healthy full term neonate is designed to withstand this period of malnutrition and dehydration. Therefore, leaving a sleeping term baby for another 4 hours after delivery before he takes his first bottle does him no harm at all. It is, however, *very* different for small-for-dates or pre-term babies, or for the infants of diabetic mothers (Chapters 11 and 15). The first feed should be with ordinary formula; there is absolutely no justification for starting with clear fluids or half strength milk. This archaic recommendation is probably based on three beliefs all of which are incorrect.

- It is worse to inhale vomit containing milk than vomit containing clear fluids: **false**. Gastric acid buffered by milk probably does less harm when inhaled than if unbuffered by water, or made more irritant by glucose solutions.
- Clear fluids are aspirated less often than milk:

false. It is just that you do not see clear fluids at laryngoscopy or autopsy!

- The infant may have a congenital malformation predisposing him to vomit, e.g. a tracheo-esophageal fistula: **false**. Firstly, because of the arguments above about vomiting, and secondly, because the diagnosis of tracheo-esophageal fistula or high obstruction should be made before the first feed is offered.

Technique of feeding

The baby should be swaddled and held closely and comfortably to the mother so that with her free hand she can hold the bottle. Touching the baby's mouth or lip with the teat will usually evoke the rooting reflex. He will turn to where the teat is and open his mouth; the teat can then be popped in. He will then suck. In bottle-feeding, he obtains milk to some extent like he does in breast-feeding, by compressing the teat with his gums and squeezing the milk in to his mouth, but since bottles do not have a 'let down reflex' (pp. 119–21) he also has to generate a vacuum in his mouth to suck the milk out of the bottle. The amount obtained per suck can be varied by varying the size of the hole in the teat. In general large holes in teats should only be used in babies with sucking problems.

A useful guideline is that if one drop of milk/second drips from the teat of an upended bottle of formula the size of the hole in the teat is appropriate.

Temperature

Traditionally, bottle milk is warmed to body temperature before feeding, but there is no need to do this, and babies take room temperature milk perfectly satisfactorily.

Frequency of feeds

Newborn babies should be demand fed, i.e. when they waken, look around and bawl for nourishment.

This is perfectly easy to arrange at home but, depressingly, more difficult in hospital. It is a totally bizarre aspect of many hospitals' routines that if a baby, either breast- or bottle-fed wakes at an inconvenient time he is given water or dextrose to shut him up till the next 4-hourly feed time is due. If a baby in the neonatal period is awake and hungry, feed him with full strength milk!

The converse is equally bizarre: shaking a baby awake just because it is 2 pm and feed time. No human being enjoys being woken unnecessarily, and adding insult to injury by force feeding him after this rude awakening does not improve things. No wonder the baby seems irritable, feeds badly, goes to sleep after only a small feed and wakes, famished, at an inconvenient time for the ward hierarchy.

Bottle-fed babies who are demand fed will usually settle in to a 3.5–4.5-hourly feeding schedule, taking 5–6 feeds per day. The ward routine must adapt to these needs.

Volume of feeds

The traditional teaching about volumes on days 1–5 and thereafter is outlined in Table 9.8. For the term baby this is only a guideline. He should be demand fed and allowed to take what he wants, which will usually average 150–180 ml/kg/day, i.e. about 90–95 ml at each of the 6 feeds. Only if there are problems with weight gain, jaundice or persistently poor feeding does it become crucial to ensure the volumes recommended in Table 9.8 are actually being taken.

TABLE 9.8 Volumes of milk to give to normal bottle-fed full term neonates

Day 1	60 ml/kg
Day 2	90 ml/kg
Day 3	120 ml/kg
Day 4	150 ml/kg
Days 7–10	180 ml/kg

ESTABLISHING BREAST-FEEDING

There are multiple factors which increase the likelihood of a woman breast-feeding satisfactorily, many of which, like the socio-economic ones, are extremely difficult to influence in the short term during pregnancy, and particularly in the crucial 48–72 hours after delivery. However, obstetricians, paediatricians and midwives can optimise the neonatal environment to make breast-feeding as easy as possible. It will be salutary for many readers to check this list against their own practice:

- encourage breast-feeding as soon after delivery as possible;
- establish rooming-in;
- do not put the baby to the breast on schedule, allow demand feeding;
- encourage the mother to feed overnight (she has to at home!);
- do not limit the time of feeding by postnatal age (e.g. 3 minutes on day 1, 5 minutes on day 2 etc.);
- do not give complementary feeds unless essential (e.g. hypoglycaemia, weight loss > 10 per cent), not just for irritability;
- do not weigh too often, or test weigh at all;
- do not offer samples of formula as a discharge gift
- ensure adequate privacy and tranquility for the learner breast-feeder;
- appoint a breast-feeding sister/counsellor.

Preparation

A mother should be advised during the antenatal period that she should breast-feed as soon as she has delivered her baby. In the past, great emphasis was put on procedures to prepare the nipples by the use of shells or manual stretching of the nipple (Hoffman's exercises). It is doubtful if these are of any benefit, and they may actually do harm (Alexander *et al.*, 1992).

Position for feeding

This is crucial. The mother should of course be comfortable and either sitting in an appropriate chair which keeps her upright and comfortable and gives her plenty of arm room, or she should adopt a similar well-supported position in bed (Fig. 9.1). An alternative is for the baby to lie beside the mother in her

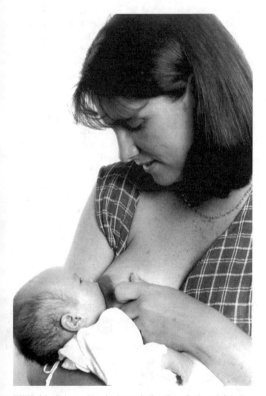

FIGURE 9.1 Sitting position for breast feeding (from Gandy and Roberton, 1987, with permission).

bed. Her environment should be calm and restful, since stress inhibits prolactin and oxytocin secretion, and thus lactation and the let down reflex. If the mother is sitting up, the baby should be lying nearly horizontal supported by her arm, or initially, while she is unsure of herself, with a cushion or pillow (Fig. 9.1). He should be comfortably and loosely swaddled. His body should be close to his mother's, and he should be facing her (i.e. front to front, not side to front); in this position the baby has to extend his neck slightly to get the nipple in to his mouth, and this leaves his lower jaw, which is the most important part of the sucking mechanism, free to move and compress the areola and the underlying lactiferous ducts.

His mother should gently stroke his lips or cheek next to her breast with a finger or with her nipple. This should evoke the rooting reflex in which the baby opens his mouth and turns to the stimulus. With a little practice, the mother can then pop her nipple in to his mouth. It is important not to try to push the baby's head on to the nipple since this upsets him and often evokes a rooting reflex from his opposite cheek so he turns away from the breast. Generalised frustration ensues. The mother should aim to insert the whole of her nipple and most of the adjacent areola into the baby's mouth. This means that his gums come into apposition over the lactiferous ducts in the sub-areolar region allowing him to squeeze the milk through the nipple into his mouth. The physical and psychological stimulus of putting the nipple in the baby's mouth should evoke the let down reflex so that milk is actively squirted in to his mouth. These are the two most important mechanisms for getting milk out of the breast, in other words during breast-feeding sucking – that is, creating a vacuum in the mouth to draw milk out of the breast – is not an important mechanism, though it is more important in bottle-feeding (p. 142).

In the first week or two, the mother, using her free hand, usually needs to support her breast in her baby's mouth and at the same time she can gently retract any part of her breast that is threatening to obstruct the baby's nose during his feed. After the first 2–3 weeks, the mother has usually acquired the knack of adopting a comfortable position for herself and her baby during a feed such that the baby's skills and strength are sufficient to allow him to fix, suckle and breathe simultaneously and successfully.

When to start

There is clearly absolutely no point in giving a breast-fed baby a first feed of clear fluid (p. 142): ideally, therefore, the first breast-feed should be undertaken in the labour ward in the first few minutes after delivery (p. 80). This is not only one of the major determinants of successful long-term lactation (Righard and Alade, 1990; Kurinij and Shiono, 1991), but by stimulating oxytocin release (p. 120) helps to contract the uterus and prevent a postpartum haemorrhage.

If the first feed cannot be given on the labour ward when the baby is bright and alert, then everyone can wait until the mother is safely ensconced in the PNW and her baby once more wakes up looking for food.

Frequency of foods

Studies on healthy mother–infant pairs in the first few days after delivery have shown that if they are both left to their own devices the baby will breast-feed up to 10–12 times a day. During these feeds the baby gets little liquid or calories but does get the immune factor rich colostrum. Since prolacatin production is turned on by nipple stimulation, frequent suckling is clearly of biological value. The message is not that babies *should* feed 10–12 times per day, but if they are awake and ready to feed they should be put to the breast. This applies not only in the first few days, but throughout lactation. Breast-fed babies in general feed more frequently than bottle-fed ones (p. 135) and in the first few days and weeks often settle into a 2.5–3.5-hourly feeding pattern. This is *normal*. The fact that this does not fit in to the preconceived hier-archical 4-hourly feeding system on a PNW is tough – on the ward! The baby should be 'rooming- in' with his mother (p. 82) and once he wakes and looks hun-gry he should be fed even if the last one was only 2 hours beforehand. Imposing the 4-hourly schedule, and topping up breast-fed babies with clear fluid, or worse, with formula, until the next feeding time is not only one of the major causes of failed lactation, but may actually increase the risk of the baby devel-oping marked jaundice, and is one of the major rea-sons why consumer groups are disaffected with the maternity services within the NHS.

Night feeds

PNW routine should always be based on the principle that a breast-feeding mother will want to be woken up to give her baby his night-time feed. Sometimes this may not be justified either because the mother is very ill or just very exhausted. It is essential though that she is given the choice. Since missing the overnight breast-feed will only happen for 1 or 2 nights, to minimise the risk of allergy (p. 132) the overnight feeds should probably be given as glucose water.

Complementary feeds

The indications for complementary feeds are given on p. 163–4. To give them should be a medical deci-sion and not based on the whim of a nurse con-fronted by an angry baby. The use of complementary feeds dramatically reduces the successful breast-feed-ing rate in a unit (Kurinij and Shiono, 1991), and is rarely if ever justified.

Free samples

Offering free samples of formulae as a discharge gift from a maternity unit should also be discouraged since it would appear to accelerate the decline in breast-feeding (Dungy *et al.*, 1992).

Duration of a feed

Most of the milk a baby is going to get comes in the first 4–6 minutes. Suckling longer than this is therefore not of nutritive value though it may have important sedative effects on the baby who will gently chomp away until he goes to sleep. There is absolutely no scientific justification for the frequent practice of starting the baby with 3 minutes at the breast on the first day, 5 minutes the next day increasing to 7 minutes and then 10 minutes. The baby even in the first day or two should be put to the breast and left there until he has finished which will usually be 6–7 minutes. Once the milk is 'in', the mother will know when he has finished because she rapidly learns the feeling when her breasts are empty. However, if he feels like sucking for more than 6–7 minutes it does no one any harm, particularly if this is to calm the baby down and prepare him for sleep.

One breast or two

In the first day or two, even when only colostrum is being produced put the baby to both breasts during a feed since apart from anything else this increases the stimulation of prolactin production. Once the baby is hungry, looking for food, and lactation is established, he will decide whether he wants one or two breasts-ful. If after the first breast is empty he has gone to sleep, the feed is over, but if he is still hungry give him the other breast. To ensure that at least one breast at a time is emptied (see p. 120 for the importance of achieving this) the mother should always alternate which breast she offers to the baby first.

Volume of feed

No mention of volume of a breast-feed is made. This is deliberate. Babies seem to be able to judge their own intake from the breast such that they grow and gain weight normally. They therefore suckle until they are 'full', and the breasts, in response to the twin stimuli of suckling and being emptied, produce enough milk of appropriate composition to supply the baby's needs (Woolridge *et al.*, 1990). If the breasts produce too much, the surplus can be sent to the milk bank in the local NNU; if they do not produce enough, or the baby does not gain weight adequately, the remedies are outlined on p. 156.

Nipple care

It is deeply enmeshed in the folklore of midwifery that frequent feeds or suckling for too long at the breast are the cause of sore nipples. This is not true (Slaven and Harvey, 1981). Sore nipples are the result of a mixture of bad luck and bad technique. There are many factors which can give women sore, red oedematous nipples which may even have petechiae on their surface. The most important is probably the position of the baby. If he fixes on the nipple rather than the areola (see above), he damages it. Other factors may be licking the nipple, or 'playing' with it by the baby. Another may be leaving dried milk on the nipple after a feed. To prevent this the mother should always carefully wash and dry her nipples after the feed. Other causes include friction from a tight bra, or chemical irritation from something applied to the nipple such as soaps or antiseptics. In all these situations the nipple soreness may progress to a crack or fissure which is extremely painful and may take several days to heal.

Some women just have bad luck, and develop these complications despite careful antenatal breast preparation and good technique during lactation, but these problems are no more common in those who indulge themselves and their babies with more frequent or more prolonged suckling. The management of sore nipples is outlined on pp. 153–5.

EXPRESSED BREAST MILK

In many situations, described above and elsewhere in this book, giving the baby milk expressed from his mother's breasts is indicated. Milk can be expressed manually with the mother holding her breasts, as shown (Fig. 9.2), and gently expressing her milk in to a sterile bowl. Most people, mothers and midwives, agree that using some form of electric breast pump such as the Egnell is much easier, and less painful. The milk collected, if it is to be used that day for the mother's own baby, can be kept in the 4°C fridge until required, but if it is being used for the milk bank, or left for longer than 24 hours before use, it should be pasteurised, checked bacteriologically and deep frozen until just before use.

MONITORING BREAST-FEEDING

There is a small definite risk of three problems in breast-fed babies: hypoglycaemia (p. 165), jaundice (p. 138) and failure to thrive (p. 162). Hypoglycaemia is a problem only in the first few days, and in full term neonates only in those who persistently feed badly and lose a lot of weight. Jaundice may occur for days or weeks, but is rarely a problem unless also associated with inadequate weight gain, but failure to thrive (that is, excessive weight loss in the first week and inadequate weight gain thereafter) can occur at any stage during breast-feeding.

The crucial monitor is thus the baby's weight. Breast-fed term babies who feed poorly for the first 3–4 days and lose >10 per cent of their birthweight should have a BM stix or Dextrostix checked daily until they are thriving, and jaundiced babies should be monitored as outlined on p. 241.

In hospital for the first few days, in addition to the weighing routines given on p. 83, the mother should note on a chart the number of times her baby goes to the breast. At home, whether the baby is 1 day or

A

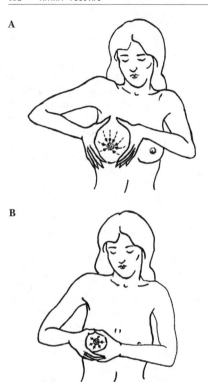

B

FIGURE 9.2 Technique for manual expression of breasts (from Gunther, 1970, with permission).

5 months old, those responsible for his care should keep a regular check to ensure that his weight gain is normal (p. 83).

If there are problems with weight gain the only way to establish the baby's intake is test weighing. In this, the baby is weighed on accurate scales just before and just after a feed without changing his clothes and nappy. The technique is, however, none too accurate and in particular has the danger that it may under-estimate at low intakes (Whitfield *et al.*, 1981). Several test weighings are probably necessary to get a feel for a baby's intake since this may vary considerably from feed to feed. Carrying out test weighing must be a last resort and only done in infants in whom failure to gain weight is becoming a serious problem. It has been shown that the anxiety provoked in a mother by this procedure, which is assessing her capacity to fulfil one of the most basic female roles, is a major inhibitor of lactation (deChateau *et al.*, 1977). Therefore, it has a distinct capacity for making things worse.

FEEDING PROBLEMS

It has to be emphasised that feeding problems must be sorted out with the mother and baby together ideally on the mother's PNW (Chapter 6). Feeding problems are emphatically *not* an indication for trans-ferring an otherwise normal baby to a NNU.

MATERNAL

For obvious reasons these are limited to the breast-feeding mother, apart from occasional problems with breast engorgement and discomfort as lactation is being suppressed in the mother who elects to bottle-feed her baby.

Nipple problems

The answer to nipple problems is, of course, preven-tion by ensuring correct positioning of the nipple in the baby's mouth during the feed and avoiding other contributory factors (p. 145). As emphasised above, frequency and duration of feeds are not a factor in the aetiology of sore nipples.

For women who have flattish nipples in the puer-perium problems are surprisingly rare since by com-pressing her areola before each feed she is usually able to push the nipple outwards, and the vigorous successful baby, by a combination of his sucking efforts and the fact that nipples become erect when stimulated, will then be able to suckle adequately.

If the nipples do become sore, the mother should be encouraged to persevere, while being meticulous with her feeding technique and with cleaning and anointing her nipples after a feed (see below), in the justified expectation that things will rapidly improve within 2–3 days. Alternatively, covering the sore nipple with a nipple shield can be helpful in this situation (Fig. 9.3). If feeding from the affected breast is too painful, or in particular if a crack or fissure develops which is not healing, then there is no alternative but to abandon feeding from that breast until healing has occurred. The baby can continue to feed from the other breast, and the affected breast must be emptied 4-hourly ideally by using an electric breast pump. The milk so obtained can then be fed to the baby by bottle or tube.

The sore inflamed nipple (p. 150) can be treated with a simple antiseptic cream such as Cetavlex to prevent infection entering, and, if the inflammation

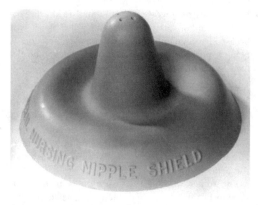

FIGURE 9.3 Nipple shield.

becomes more marked 0.5 per cent hydrocortisone cream is also helpful. Sprays, alcohols and tincture of Benzoin are extremely painful on raw tissue and should never be used.

Swallowed maternal blood from a cracked nipple is probably the most common cause of haematemesis and melaena in the neonate (pp. 263–5).

Breast engorgement

When the milk first comes in, the mother's breasts may become full very quickly and become so tight and engorged that by the time the next feed is due the nipple and areola just cannot be taken into the infant's mouth. This is managed by expressing 20–30 ml of breast milk, most comfortably by using a breast pump; this slackens the breasts sufficiently to enable the baby to fix satisfactorily on to the nipple and thereafter feed normally. In the vast majority of cases, engorgement is a transient early phenomenon and the mother's supply settles down to meet demand within the first week or two. If it does not, she may always need to express a small amount of milk before the start of a feed.

The discomfort caused by engorgement in the first few days may be so intense in some women that it merits treatment with conventional analgesics. In some, the build-up of pressure results in extravasation of milk in a segment of the breast, into the breast tissue itself. The mother may then become pyrexial, the breast becomes red and tender, and a mass may be palpable in one lobule; this is the condition of acute mastitis. Treatment is to give analgesics and regularly empty the breast 4-hourly. However, since manual expression is extremely painful, a breast pump is essential, and there is always a distinct risk of breast abscess developing. If there is any doubt about infection, antistaphylococcal antibiotics should be given.

Breast abscess

This is usually secondary to acute mastitis, but can develop from superficial infection near the areola, particularly if cord care has been poor (p. 85), or staphylococcal infection is present elsewhere in the baby or in the mother. The mother is febrile, toxic, with an acutely tender inflamed breast lobule. She needs antibiotics and antipyretics/analgesics, and lactation should normally be suppressed.

Inadequate milk production

Many women give up breast-feeding for this reason, yet careful studies of women in this situation suggests that their lactation is adequate (Hellervik-Linquist *et al.*, 1991) and they should therefore be encouraged to persevere. If, however, inadequate milk production is diagnosed on the basis of poor weight gain and inadequate intake documented on test weighing the baby, then the first thing to do is to increase deliberately the frequency of suckling to 2–3-hourly. The increased nipple stimulation, by increasing prolactin secretion, will probably increase milk production. Check that the mother is having an adequate fluid and calorie intake. If this does not work a trial of metoclopramide can be undertaken. This drug increases prolactin production by hypothalamic stimulation. If this does not work, and the baby is still not thriving, then the mother has to come to terms either with giving up breast-feeding or committing herself to long-term complementary feeds (p. 163) in the usually forlorn hope that her own lactation will improve. Once there has been a problem with deficient lactation the mother–infant pair require careful paediatric supervision in the future to ensure that the baby continues to gain weight adequately.

Too much milk

Milk may come out of the contralateral breast when the baby is sucking; it may drip out of both breasts between feeds; and/or the woman may have persisting problems with engorgement. Leaking milk can be absorbed with pads, and breast engorgement can be treated by emptying some milk out before the start of a feed. In general, these problems settle down with the passage of time since physiologically (see above) milk production is geared to consumption.

Suppression of lactation

If, for some reason, suppression is necessary, nothing need be done. In most women, in the absence of suckling, prolactin secretion rapidly falls off and the milk production stops, with very little breast discomfort or engorgement. It is nevertheless common to use bromocriptine to suppress prolactin production. The dose is 2.5 mg b.d. for a fortnight.

Breast-feeding and cancer

The relationship between breast-feeding and subsequent breast cancer is not clarified, though if there is an influence, it is that the woman who has breastfed has a decreased risk of breast cancer (Vorherr, 1979).

Rarities

Women with unilateral absence of a breast or who have had a mastectomy can try to feed from their single breast, though for obvious reasons the volume produced may be inadequate. Rare women, despite apparently structurally normal breasts, fail to lactate, presumably due to end-organ insensitivity to the hormonal stimuli. The diagnosis of breast malignancy late in pregnancy or after delivery is a contraindication to breast-feeding since immediate maternal treatment is imperative. Women who have had augmentation mammoplasty can breast-feed, since the augmentation procedure is carried out behind the normal breast tissue which is left undamaged by the procedure. Women who have had reduction mammoplasty, however, should not breast-feed, since the procedure usually disconnects the areola from the underlying structures, and milk flow is not possible.

BABY PROBLEMS

Baby problems are also more common in breast-fed babies; however they are not unknown in bottle-fed babies.

Baby not feeding

A common problem is that the baby refuses to wake up and, in particular, breast-feed at the appropriate time, or contrary to what has been said above he is one of those (normal) breast-feeding babies who decided he wants only five feeds per day.

It is, of course, essential to ensure that the 'unwilling-to-feed' baby is not ill, and in particular to examine him carefully to exclude dyspnoea, congenital heart disease, dysmorphic syndromes (e.g. Down's syndrome) or some primary neuromuscular disorder (pp. 255–7) and to make sure that his mouth is normal. It is embarrassing to miss a cleft palate. It is important to exclude hypoglycaemia by Dextrostix estimation, and if there is any suspicion of infection (pp. 293–7) appropriate investigations should be carried out.

If these problems can be excluded, and this is usually very easy to do, three important things must be remembered.

- The normal full term baby, designed to be breast-fed, is not 'expecting' any calories in the first 24–48 hours till his mother's milk comes in. Some just decide to doze through this period.
- Normal babies cannot tell the time particularly if they are asleep, and so they do not wake on a 4-hourly schedule; if they are shaken awake, they tend to be grumpy and singularly unenthusiastic about feeding.
- So long as a baby is gaining weight normally he is getting enough to eat.

If the non-feeding baby is a normally grown full term one who is in fact behaving entirely normally, nothing needs to be done irrespective of whether he is breast- or bottle-fed other than to 'demand feed'. That is, wait for him to wake up, even if it takes 5–6 hours, whereupon he will feed and thrive. The only possible drawback with this is that it does not give the mother optimal breast stimulation, and although this could in theory compromise her ultimate lactation performance, this is rarely if ever a problem. However, if the baby's refusal to feed really is outside the normal range alluded to above, then the most common causes are:

- prematurity (p. 186);
- the aftermath of a difficult delivery, e.g. Kielland's forceps;
- sedation from intrapartum or antenatal drug therapy, e.g. narcotics, general anaesthesia;
- sedation from drugs in the breast milk.

In the second and third groups all that usually needs to be done is to wait patiently, and in 24–48 hours the baby improves his feeding spontaneously. If he received a narcotic analgesic intrapartum, it is worth testing the effect of a single dose of naloxone (0.1 mg/kg i.m. × 1). In rare cases, it may be necessary to gave these babies one or two tube feeds before they suckle satisfactorily, and if the mother's intention is to breast-feed her baby he should be given her breast milk down the nasogastric tube.

If the problem is due to the fourth cause this probably means that unless the mother's therapy can be discontinued, which is not usually possible, breast-feeding is contraindicated. If none of the above is the cause, and the feeding problem persists, careful re-evaluation to exclude some underlying neurological or muscular disorder is indicated but in general a few tube feeds and passage of time results in a complete cure!

Crying

There are many causes for babies crying, notably pain, discomfort usually from a loaded nappy, and boredom, as well as hunger. Experienced nurses, mothers and even GPs or paediatricians can usually tell which is which. If the diagnosis is hunger, the appropriate treatment is food, even if the baby was only fed 2–2.5 hours previously. As expressed above, feeding this frequently is often required in breast-fed infants. If the crying baby shows no enthusiasm for feeding and is clean and dry, then he needs to be comforted by cuddling, by being walked around with, and being talked to. Eventually he will either go to sleep or calm down enough to feed. If he does not, then it is just possible that there is something wrong, and in the persistently screaming baby one must exclude comparatively occult but very painful conditions, e.g. acute otitis media, intussusception, bone and joint sepsis, incarcerated hernia – though clearly these are all rare in the neonatal period. In the neonatal period persistent crying usually responds to cuddling and/or food. It is, however, commonly believed that crying in a baby is due to wind (though this is probably untrue – (see below) and/or can only be treated by a complementary feed of some non-maternal fluid such as water or dextrose (though this is only rarely true).

Wind

In a bottle-fed baby, it is inevitable that, as the baby sucks down the millk, he will take in some air, either because the mother has allowed the meniscus in the bottle to lie across the hole in the teat, or just because at the end of the bottle-feed, it is impossible to slurp down the last few millilitres without taking in some air as well. After the feed, the mother sits her baby upright, hopefully in such a position that the stomach gas bubble lies underneath the oesophageal hiatus and then by rubbing or patting his back induces the bubble to burst upwards. The resulting burp is regarded with the accolade of approval by all within earshot and the baby is then expected to sleep.

The female breast is better designed than a milk bottle and does not contain air! The breast-fed baby therefore should, and probably does, swallow less air during a feed. Nevertheless, he is still submitted to the same assault on his back in the expectation that he will burp, and he probably will do, since we all, if healthy, have some gas in our stomach.

Since adults with various forms of non-specific abdominal pain frequently find relief, if not pleasure in breaking wind, there is a deeply ingrained belief that one of the causes of a baby screaming as outlined above, and apparently in pain, is wind, probably having escaped beyond the stomach and passing distally through the bowel. One corollary to this belief is that wind, and therefore the screaming, can be prevented by vigorously pounding over the infant's spine immediately after a feed to release surplus gases from his stomach before they enter the small intestines. A little thought should convince us that this is absolute nonsense, and merely results in mutual maternal and neonatal exhaustion. I would not dare to suggest that infants should not be 'winded', but after a feed the infant should be sat upright lying slightly forward over one of his mother's hands, while she gently rubs or pats his back with the other. If nothing comes up after 2–3 minutes, the procedure should be abandoned, and the baby allowed to sleep; if he is still restless, another cause, specifically hunger, should be considered.

Colic

There is no doubt at all that some babies have episodes in which they scream, go puce, and by their behaviour, in particular the way they draw up their legs, give everyone the very strong impression that they are in pain. It is also clear that some babies begin to show this pattern in the neonatal period, and many of the neonates who resist all the above ruses to control their irritability and screaming often go on to develop more obvious features of colic by 2–3 months of age. Unfortunately, we have no idea what colic is due to, but it is definitely *not* wind, hunger, food allergy or intolerance. The problem has to be explained sympathetically to the parents who devise a multitude of tricks to induce their screaming baby to sleep. Fortunately, the condition spontaneously resolves by 3–4 months of age. Various anticolic medicines have been used, and gripe waters of old are still used, and probably owe their benefit to the fact that they are sedatives due to their high alcohol content. Dicyclomine (Merbentyl) is a successful drug proven to be effective in prospective trials, but a cautionary note has crept in since the report of hypersensitivity reactions in a very small number of infants following its use. Since these infants were not seriously ill, and these are the only adverse sequelae reported from what must have been millions of administered doses worldwide, the drug should still have a place in the management of infantile colic (Illingworth, 1985).

Poor weight gain/persisting hunger

When evaluating these problems in the neonatal period, remember that by far the most common cause is an inadequate caloric intake. Nevertheless, before assuming this, it is essential to take a careful history and to examine the baby thoroughly to exclude some organic cause for failure to thrive such as diarrhoea, heart disease or some dysmorphic syndrome. However, if the history and examination are negative, test weighing confirms an inadequate intake and despite implementing all the ruses outlined above the baby still fails to thrive, there does come a time when it is clear that the problem cannot be solved by increasing the number of breast-feeds, cuddling the baby, maternal metoclopramide and so on, and some extra source of liquid and/or calories is the only way to solve the feeding problem, calm a

hungry crying baby, or get him to gain weight. This
time has come:

(a) With persisting failure to settle a crying fractious
baby over a short period of time. This clearly has
many different interpretations depending on
many variables. Examples would be a baby who
has gone to an empty or virtually empty breast
three times in 4–5 hours and is obviously still
famished. Another is a baby needing 2-hourly
feeds but not settling satisfactorily after them nor
gaining weight; it does *not* mean a baby who is
gaining weight, feeding well 2–3-hourly, then
sleeping and waking refreshed for more food;
that baby needs his next normal breast-feed.

(b) If the weight loss exceeds 10 per cent (p. 83), there
is a temperature (dehydration fever, p. 165), hypoglycaemia (p. 165) or severe jaundice (p. 243).

(c) In the presence of nipple or engorgement problems, when only one breast is being used, and as
a result the baby is underfed. In many such
babies the extra feed can be a bottle-feed of the
mother's milk pumped from the affected breast.

(d) If a baby persistently loses weight after 4–5 days
of age or fails to gain weight after 6–7 days of
age, particularly if there are other signs that the
baby has a poor intake, e.g. fitful, hungry, a poor
intake on a test weighing.

(e) When the mother is demoralised, calming her
baby with a few bottle-feeds and giving her eight
hours sleep may transform the situation and
allow normal lactation to be established afterwards.

Since one of the purported advantages of breast-feeding is the reduction in the incidence of cows' milk
protein induced malabsorption, and there is the possibility that this syndrome may be induced even by
one or two cows' milk formula feeds in the neonatal
period, the conventional wisdom is to give groups
(a)–(c) above, and probably even group (d) and (e),

the additional feeds as 5 or 10 per cent dextrose which is non-allergenic, slakes thirst and does give some calories (20 and 40 kCal/100 ml respectively). In most cases in groups (a),(b),(c) and (e) no more than 3–4 such feeds will be needed to tide the mother and baby pair over the crisis, and normal breast-feeding can then be resumed. However, if (d) remains a problem calories and protein are needed, and this means milk.

Extra feeds in any situations can be given either as a complementary feed (i.e. the baby goes to both breasts and is then offered a bottle till satisfied) or a supplementary feed (i.e. an entire breast-feed is omitted and replaced by an appropriate volume of bottle-feed).

A short period of complementary and supplementary feeding with bottle milk is often justified in groups (d) and (e), but rather than giving the mother's lactation time to improve, in fact this line of management often proves counterproductive (see p. 148), since the decreased suckling at the breast which results, decreases prolactin and thus decreases milk production. The ultradetermined mother can persist with extra complementary feeds or use some of the devices such as the Lactaid in which a fine plastic cannula connected to a bag of milk is placed in the sucking baby's mouth so that as well as getting milk from both sources (breast plus Lactaid) he stimulates his mother's nipples and hopefully prolactin and breast milk production. However, if the baby's failure to thrive at the breast does not respond to reasonable attempts to improve matters over 3–4 days, given the minimal disadvantages of using formula feeds, I would advise the mother to give up breast-feeding and put the baby on the bottle. The look of relief and gratitude that usually spreads across the face of the mother who has had the burden of making that decision taken from her, and can now relax into 4-hourly bottle-feeds, usually vindicates my decision.

Dehydration fever

If a baby on the first week of life develops a fever, the two most likely and important causes are infection (p. 295), or overheating due to some defect in the environmental control such as lying a heavily swaddled term baby in direct sunlight and alongside a radiator which is on full blast. In the first few days of life, if these are excluded, the febrile baby who is clinically well but is feeding poorly and has lost 10 per cent or more of his birthweight may be suffering from dehydration.

Hypoglycaemia

Hypoglycaemia (pp. 277–9) may occasionally occur on the third or fourth day even in a full term normally grown baby if he has been breast-feeding unusually badly. It can and should be prevented by checking the blood glucose by BM stix or Dextrostix (p. 185) and responding accordingly (p. 279).

Gastroenterological symptoms

Vomiting, diarrhoea, abdominal distension and jaundice all require evaluation in their own right (Chapters 17, 18); they are rarely due to feeding problems, though jaundice is frequently associated with breast-feeding. I would emphasise that such symptoms should never be managed by changing the milk given to the baby.

REFERENCES

Alexander, J.M., Grant, A.M. and Campbell, M.J. (1992). Randomised controlled trial of breast shells and Hoffman's exercises for inverted and non-protractile nipples. *British Medical Journal* **304**, 1030–1032.

American Academy of Pediatrics (1992). The use of whole cow's milk in infancy. *Pediatrics* **89**, 1105–1109.

deChateau, P., Holmberg, H., Jakobsson, K. and Winberg, J. (1977). A study of factors promoting and inhibiting lactation. *Developmental Medicine and Child Neurology* **19**, 575–584.

Dewey, K.G., Heinig, M.J., Nommsen, L.A., Peersen, J.M. and Lönnerdal, B. (1992). Growth of breast-fed and formula-fed infants from 0–18 months: the DARLING study. *Pediatrics* **89**, 1035–1041.

Dungy, C.I., Christensen-Szalansk, J., Losch, M. and Russel, D. (1992). Effect of discharge samples on duration of breast-feeding. *Pediatrics* **90**, 233–237.

Glasier, A. and McNeilly, A.S. (1990). *Baillière's Clinical Endocrinology & Metabolism*, vol. 4, pp. 379–395.

Hellervik-Linquist, C., Hofvander, Y. and Sjölin, S. (1991). Studies on perceived breast milk insufficiency. *Acta Paediatrica Scandinavica* **80**, 297–303.

HMSO (1993). *The Sleeping Position of Infants and Cot Death.* HMSO, London.

Illingworth, R.S. (1985). Infantile colic revisited. *Archives of Disease in Childhood* **60**, 981–985.

Kramer, M.S. (1988). Does breast-feeding protect against atopic disease?: biology, methodology and a golden jubilee of controversy. *Journal of Pediatrics* **112**, 181–190.

Kurinij, N. and Shiono, P.H. (1991). Early formula sup-plementation of breast-feeding. *Pediatrics* **88**, 745–750.

Richard, L. and Alade, M.O. (1990). Effect of delivery room routines on success of first breast-feed. *Lancet* **336**, 1105–1107.

Savilahti, E., Tainio, V.M., Salmenperä, L., Siimes, M.A. and Perheentupa, J. (1987). Prolonged exclusive breast-feed-ing and heredity as determinants of infantile atopy. *Archives of Diseases in Childhood* **62**, 269–273.

Short, R.V., Lewis, P.R. Renfree, M.B. and Shaw, G. (1991). Contraceptive effects of extended lactational amen-orrhoea: beyond the Bellagio consensus. *Lancet* **337**, 715–717.

Slaven, S. and Harvey, D.R. (1981). Unlimited suckling time improves breast-feeding. *Lancet* **i**, 392–393.

Vorherr, H. (1979). Pregnancy and lactation in relation to breast cancer risk. *Seminars in Perinatology* **3**, 299–311.

Whitfield, M.F., Kay, R. and Stevens, S. (1981). Validity of routine clinical test weighing as a meaasure of the intake of breast-fed infants. *Archives of Disease in Childhood* **56**, 919–921.

Woolridge, M.W., Ingram, J.C. and Baum, J.D. (1990). Do changes in the pattern of breast usage alter the baby's nutri-ent intake. *Lancet* **336**, 395–397.

FURTHER READING

Freed, D.L.J. (1984). *The Health Hazards of Milk.* Baillière Tindall, London.

Gunther, M. (1970). *Infant Feeding.* Methuen & Co. Ltd., London.

Lucas, A. (1992). Infant feeding. Part I & II. In: *Textbook of Neonatology,* 2nd Ed. Ed. Roberton, N.R.C. Churchill Livingstone, London, Edinburgh, pp. 251–277.

10

CRITERIA FOR ADMISSION TO NEONATAL UNITS

—

INTRODUCTION

A neonatal unit should now be an integral part of all maternity hospitals. These neonatal units may take on the care of all critically ill neonates born in the hospital, or may have a system of referring the sickest and smallest of their patients to regional intensive care units. It has been shown that for neonatal intensive care, as with all aspects of medical care dealing with seriously ill patients, concentrating resources in a small number of centres is not only more economical, but also creates centres of experience and, thereby, expertise and excellence.

With the increasing interest in the care of ill low birthweight neonates in the 1960s and 1970s the number of babies admitted to these neonatal intensive care units steadily increased, so that by the mid to late 1970s in England and Wales an average of 20 per cent of all neonates were admitted, with some hospitals admitting up to 40 per cent. This level of admission was clearly absurd and is no longer necessary (if indeed it ever was) for five reasons:

- Increasing the number of babies in the NNU increases the risks among them of *nosocomial infection.*
- It was based on *misinterpretation of the data* on which

were, and which were not, high-risk patients.

- Advances in obstetric and neonatal care have now made *safe the management on PNW* of many conditions which in the past were thought to merit NNU admission.
- It *misuses those facilities* which are nationally in short supply, but are desperately needed for the care of very ill, very low birthweight neonates.
- It causes unjustified *mother–child separation.*

RISKS OF NOSOCOMIAL INFECTION

For obvious reasons, the NNU of any maternity hospital contains the sickest patients in the hospital, some of whom have been admitted with serious infectious disease, and many of whom, because of the instrumentation and monitoring inherent in intensive care are colonised with unpleasant, hospital derived, antibiotic resistant and often Gram negative organisms. It is the unit in the hospital, therefore, where, despite meticulous techniques to minimise infection, serious infectious disease still occurs, sometimes in epidemic form. Furthermore, the busier and more crowded any intensive care unit is, the more likely it is that there will be nosocomial spread of infection. Therefore, admitting a neonate unnecessarily to a busy NNU not only puts him at risk from infection, but by adding one more to the crowd increases the risk of infection not only for himself, but for all the other babies in the unit.

It also has to be stressed over and over again (pp. 217–9) that sick babies, and in particular the nursing and medical staff in NNUs, are colonised with hospital acquired bacteria, and are a much greater microbiological hazard to the neonate than his parents and siblings, no matter how grubby and unsavoury they may appear to be.

MISINTERPRETATION OF DATA

Many admissions to NNUs in the past were unjustified. For example, admitting babies delivered by the breech or caesarean section was based on misinterpretation of obstetric data. Although infants delivered by caesarean or breech *are* more likely to get ill than normal vaginal deliveries, this is either because of the reason for the caesarean section, because such deliveries are more often premature or because the neonate has some problem apparent immediately after birth. If infants delivered by caesarean section or the breech are pink, vigorous, mature and asymptomatic at 10 minutes of age, they do just as well as spontaneous vertex deliveries (Campbell, *et al.* 1983) and the same type of false logic applies to the routine admission of all twin deliveries.

Some admissions were also due to incorrect diagnoses often made by nursing staff in an era when 24 hour paediatric input into neonatal care was unusual. For example, traumatic cyanosis (p. 251) would be confused with central cyanosis, jitteriness with fits, or having a rhesus negative mother without antibodies with a rhesus negative mother *with* antibodies. Such problems should now be a thing of the past, as should some of the totally incomprehensive reasons for admitting neonates to an NNU such as feeding problems or maternal illness. Sticking babies who are feeding badly in an NNU away from their mothers is a singularly inappropriate way of solving their mutual problems; taking the baby away from some woman with steroid dependent asthma or on anticonvulsants in the false belief that the drugs or the illness might affect the neonate is not only medically unjustifiable (Chapter 3) but also cruel.

ADVANCES IN OBSTETRIC AND NEONATAL CARE

Improved intrapartum anaesthesia and the increased use of epidural anaesthesia for caesarean section means that infants delivered this way are no longer affected by the aftermath of a prolonged and neo-natally sedating general anaesthetic. Sophisticated antenatal management of maternal diabetes now means that their infants can be safely managed with their mothers on a PNW (Chapter 15). Improved understanding of the management of pre-term neonates, SFD neonates and the use of phototherapy for jaundice has enabled neonates with these prob-lems to be managed on a PNW rather than taken in to the NNU (Chapters 11,17).

MISUSE OF FACILITIES

The nurse trained in neonatal intensive care is at pre-sent one of the most scarce and thus valuable com-modities in the NHS. Nursing levels in many British neonatal intensive care units, particularly at night, at weekends or at times of staff sickness or annual leave, are seriously below those recommended by the pro-fessional bodies. The talents and experience of such nurses must be concentrated on those babies who need them most, and not diluted by having to care for babies who not only do not need to be in an NNU, but who would be, in any case, much better cared for by getting individual attention from highly motivated and skilful nurses – their mothers.

MOTHER–CHILD SEPARATION

As the initial obsession for this subject has calmed down, it has become clear that some of the more extreme views expressed in the mid-1970s were unjustified; nevertheless, certain assertions have stood the test of time and re-evaluation (Richards, 1992).

- Except in extreme circumstances the deleterious psychological and developmental sequelae of mother–child separation in the early neonatal period are transient and fully recoverable. Nevertheless, even these should be avoided if possible, and this will also reduce the small minority of cases in whom early mother–baby separation does cause bigger and more long-term problems.

- Putting the baby to the breast in the first hour is not only enjoyable (probably for both mother and baby), but is one of the major determinants of successful long-term lactation (p. 147).

- In general, mothers much prefer having their babies with them, and the reverse is probably also the case. To deny each this pleasure without some excellent reason is medically unjustified and socially cruel.

- Mothers' concepts of malformations in their babies are much worse than the realities. Unless a baby has a malformation which is life-threatening, or needs urgent investigation, medical care or surgery, he should stay on the PNW with his mother.

CONCLUSION

For all these reasons, the criteria for admitting babies to the NNU should be just two.

1. Birthweight < 1.70–1.80 kg:

   Such babies rarely nipple-feed adequately and often have problems sustaining their body temperature in the environmental temperature of a PNW.

2. Illness:

   Of the sort that in an older infant would probably necessitate admission to hospital from home. In babies over 2.0 kg with such illnesses,

90 per cent are apparent at birth or within the next 10–15 minutes. The remaining 10 per cent have conditions such as congenital intestinal obstruction, late onset sepsis, marked jaundice, many types of seizure and most inborn errors of metabolism which, by their very nature, must present after the first few minutes or hours of life, and would not be prevented by routinely admitting many normal babies immediately after delivery (Campbell *et al.*, 1983). Minor illnesses which in an older baby could be managed by the GP at home or by out-patient visits can be very successfully managed on a postnatal ward.

Our experience in Cambridge over the last 10 years, has consistently shown that using these criteria about 6–6.5 per cent of all live births need to be admitted to the NNU, and that in infants over 2.00 kg and in particularly over 2.50 kg, NNU admission should be the exception rather than the rule (Table 10.1).

TABLE 10.1 Admission to the Neonatal Unit, Rosie Maternity Hospital Cambridge, 1992 (Inborn babies only)

Birthweight (kg)	Number born	Number admitted	Per cent
< 1.00	28	28	100
1.00–1.499	42	42	100
1.50–1.999	57	43	75
2.0–2.499	196	52	27
≥ 2.50	4219	134	3.1
Total	4581	300	6.5

In the following chapters, I will outline the management of the smaller babies on a PNW, and describe the management of the minor medical problems which can be coped with on a PNW, in a GP maternity unit or at home.

REFERENCES

Campbell, D.M., Gandy, G.M. and Roberton, N.R.C. (1983). Which babies need admission to Special Care Baby Units? In: *Parent–Baby Attachment in Premature Infants.* Davis, J.A., Richards, M.P.M. and Roberton, N.R.C. Croom Helm, London and Canberra, pp. 67–85.

Richards, M.P.M. (1992). Psychological aspects of neonatal care. In: *Textbook of Neonatology.* 2nd Ed. Ed. Roberton, N.R.C. Churchill Livingstone, London, Edinburgh, pp. 29–42.

11

CARE OF SMALL BABIES ON A POSTNATAL WARD

—

ORGANISATION

Most of this section applies to babies who will be kept in hospital on a PNW, but many such babies will by 7–10 days of age be discharged home and the general principles of care there are also set out in this chapter.

CRITERIA FOR ADMISSION

As outlined in the previous chapter, a healthy, newborn baby weighing 1.70–2.50 kg, be he a twin, small-for-dates (SFD) or just pre-term, can be cared for on a postnatal ward (PNW) with his mother. From our own review of such babies in Cambridge it is clear that the clinical decision to transfer such a baby to a PNW can be made immediately after delivery by midwives or SHOs in the labour ward, and that their assessments are safe and accurate. A small number of 32–36 weeks gestation infants may develop some kind of mild respiratory disease for the first time after 1–2 hours of age. They can then be transferred to the NNICU without any detriment. There is no evidence that subsequent admission to the NNICU of small babies initially admitted to a PNW is ever caused by a condition which would have been prevented by routine admission post delivery, nor that the prognosis or outcome of the condition was compromised by it developing on a PNW rather than on the NNICU (Whitby *et al.*, 1982).

CARE OF THE MOTHERS OF LOW BIRTHWEIGHT INFANTS

Babies weighing 1.70–2.50 kg even if asymptomatic often need to stay in hospital for 10–14 days, and it is often stated that caring for them on a PNW will fail because their mothers will not be prepared or able to stay in with them. Although we do see this occasionally, particularly with babies or twins who need 14 days or more on the PNW, it is the exception rather than the rule. We find that if we tell the mothers the truth, namely that it is in the best interests of both them and their baby to stay in the hospital together for this period of time, the offer is eagerly accepted. Incarceration of the mother in the hospital is reduced to a minimum by discharging the baby as soon as possible (p. 193) and adopting a liberal attitude to letting the mother go out for an hour or two to go home, to do some shopping, or have a meal with her husband.

In the rare case where the mother does decide that she must go home, and in particular if the baby is only going to need to stay in hospital for a few more days, we would keep him on the PNW nursery and have him looked after by the PNW nurses since this leaves the NNICU to concentrate on what it is there for, and spares the baby exposure to the increased risk of nosocomial infection inherent in admission to the NNICU (p. 169).

STAFFING THE PNW

Keeping 32–36 weeks' gestation babies, SFD babies or twins on a PNW does not mean abandoning them to their fate away from medical care and supervision. The paediatric input into such, albeit healthy, neonates is greater than that required on a PNW for a normal 3.5 kg, 40 weeks' gestation baby. This extra input is justified because care on a PNW is the optimal care for the 1.70–2.50 kg neonate.

However, the paediatrician's role is primarily in the organisation of such a unit, and in a willingness, if the baby stays in for 10–14 days, to check him regularly. In addition, the paediatrician will have to devise and ensure the implementation of routines for the prevention and/or recognition of problems like hypoglycaemia in SFD neonates (p. 184) and for the management of conditions which are more likely to develop in a pre-term neonate than a full term one, for example feeding problems (p. 158) or jaundice (p. 238 et. seq.).

In Cambridge, in the PNW on which these small babies are cared for by their mothers, the nursing staff is the same as on any PNW, though in order to get more experience in the supervision of these small babies the sisters stay longer than they do when they are rotated to other units in the maternity hospital. Overnight we also make sure that the nurse on duty is a fully trained staff midwife, though she is usually on her own with the help of a nursing auxiliary. The nurse manager of the NNICU also supervises this ward.

ROUTINE MEDICAL CARE OF SMALL BABIES

The care of all these babies on the labour ward is identical to that described for term babies in Chapter 6. Particular emphasis, however, must be placed on keeping them warm (see below), since they cool off more easily than larger babies. They must receive vitamin K (see below), since pre-term infants have low levels of most clotting factors. In both the labour ward and PNW the other aspects of neonatal care such as umbilical cord care (p. 85), weighing (p. 83), examination (Chapter 7), screening (Chapter 8) and family visiting (p. 85), are exactly the same as for term babies. It is important to emphasise that 'rooming-in', i.e. having the baby or babies in a cot by the mother's bedside, is also a routine.

OBSERVATIONS

These babies, particularly if pre-term rather than SFD, may develop mild respiratory illness in the first few hours of life even though they were completely asymptomatic in the labour ward. For this reason they should have their temperature, pulse and respiration recorded on admission to the PNW and 6 hourly during the next 24 hours. Thereafter, daily observations are all that are required. Apnoea monitoring is not indicated; if it *is* felt to be necessary in an individual baby, he should be transferred to a NNU.

TEMPERATURE CONTROL

Having a smaller body mass, small babies are more prone to hypothermia both in the labour ward (p. 73) and in the PNW. Great care does need to be taken to prevent this. The most effective way to do it is to keep the baby clothed and wearing a hat. He can and should be nursed in a cot, and I have no doubt that the normal 1.80 kg baby can be cot nursed from the moment of birth. The chart (Fig. 11.1) shows that these babies in a cot need to be in a warmer than average ward (say 22.5–25°C) for the first few days, but by 10 days can usually be safely managed in a 21°C room. Our experience is that these temperatures are not uncomfortable for the staff or parents, and that even in the first few days an environmental temperature of 22.5°C is usually adequate for a fully clothed and swaddled 2.00 kg baby.

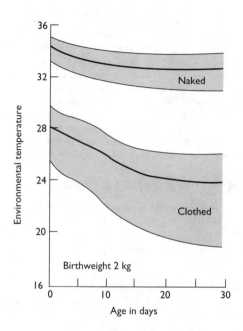

FIGURE 11.1 The optimal environmental temperature at which to nurse a normal 2.00 kg baby so that his temperature stays normal. In the top part of the figure is the data for a naked baby, and the bottom part the data for a clothed one. The solid line represents the optimal temperature and the shaded area the acceptable range of environmental temperatures within which the baby will keep his temperature at 37°C without having to expend energy to generate heat (from Hey, 1971).

COLD BABIES

If one of these small babies is found to have a temperature of 35–35.5°C it is usually just after admission to the PNW from the labour ward. The correct thing to do is to examine the baby and to check that he is otherwise well. If he is, clothe him (including a hat), wrap him in a sheet and cover him in two blankets, and place him in a warm environment near a radiator, under a radiant warmer, or in a 25°C nursery – and check his temperature 30 minutes and 60 minutes later. If it comes up to 37°C, as it usually does, no further treatment is required. If it does not, or if a baby who has been on a PNW for some time becomes hypothermic, it is safer to admit him to the NNICU for evaluation and re-warming. Do not put cold babies on a hot water bottle, or on heating pads in the cot, since if they are too hot, the baby cannot wriggle free and can only too easily be burned.

THE NORMAL PRE-TERM INFANT

It is now generally accepted that the majority of infants at a gestation of 32–36 weeks or B.Wt. 1.80–2.50 kg can be cared for on a PNW by and with their mothers, with a little help from the nursing staff (p. 175, Whitby *et al.*, 1982). In addition, many babies of this gestation can be cared for on the PNW with their mothers after they have had a spell of 2–3 days in the neonatal unit for some short-lived problem such as transient tachypnoea of the newborn or the aftermath of mild birth asphyxia.

WEIGHT CHANGES

In general these are no different from those in term babies, that is, up to 10 per cent of the body weight may normally be lost in the first 4–5 days, after which body weight should increase at roughly 10–15 g/kg/24 hrs. In the more premature babies nearer 32 weeks and 1.70 kg it may take 6–8 days before their weight begins to increase.

MEDICAL PROBLEMS

Prevention of infection

The more premature an infant, the more susceptible he is to infection since he has missed out on some of the transplacental infusion of maternal IgG. Nevertheless, the healthy 32–36 week neonate on a PNW will come to no harm so long as the precautions outlined in Chapter 16 for prevention of infection in term babies are carried out. The presentation and management of infection in such babies is outlined in Chapters 16 and 19.

Jaundice
(Chapter 17)

Premature babies are more prone to jaundice than mature ones. However, the management in the healthy premature infant is no different from that outlined in Chapter 17 except that phototherapy should be instituted at slightly lower levels than in the term baby (Fig. 17.2).

Hypoglycaemia
(p. 277)

Pre-term babies are more likely to develop hypoglycaemia (blood glucose < 1.5 mmol/l) than term babies and should have Dextrostix measurements 8 hourly through the first 48 hours, and at any time after this if there are problems with feeding. However, so long as feeding is progressing satisfactorily on a PNW, hypoglycaemia, in our experience, is very rare.

THE NORMAL SMALL-FOR-DATES BABY

The definition of smallness-for-dates is given on p. 7. Our own experience has shown that it is only babies whose birthweight is below the 3rd centile who merit the special assessment and supervision outlined in this section (Jones and Roberton, 1986). Physicians of a more nervous disposition may wish to include in such surveillance all babies whose birthweights are below the 5th or 10th centile. However, I would encourage the reader to use only the 3rd centile (Table 2.1, Chapter 2).

In general, SFD babies < 1.70 kg should be admitted to the NNICU almost irrespective of gestation, since they are very prone to develop hypoglycaemia in the first 24–48 hours, but those bigger than this can be kept on a PNW with their mother and their care is described below. This section, as with the previous one on pre-term babies, is dealing with infants of birthweight 1.70–2.50 kg. However, since the 3rd centile at 35–36 weeks is about 1.80 kg, the babies described in this section are in general mature. It is an old adage that babies act their age and not their weight, and so the behaviour and abilities of SFD babies, particularly where sucking and feeding is concerned are those of a term baby.

ASSESSMENT OF SFD BABIES

The birthweight of all newborn babies should be checked against a birthweight for gestational age list (Table 2.1); those below the 3rd centile should be managed as SFD.

Scrawny babies (Clifford's syndrome)

In addition to babies below the 3rd centile, the scrawny, often postmature baby with Clifford's syndrome deserves special attention. These babies although commonly above the 3rd or even the 10th centile for weight, and usually having a normal length and head circumference for their gestation, have a characteristic scrawny appearance with little subcutaneous fat. They were presumably intended to be 4.0 kg term babies until intrauterine growth retardation took over. They look wide eyed and alert, should be recognised clinically, and included in the screening procedures for SFD neonates since they have also suffered marked intrauterine growth retardation and are at risk from hypoglycaemia.

ANXIETY ABOUT SMALL-FOR-DATES BABIES

Perinatal anxiety about this group of babies centres on four main areas: intrauterine death, intrapartum asphyxia, congenital malformations and neonatal hypoglycaemia, all adding up to an increased perinatal mortality. Our own experience is that such anxiety is, by and large, unfounded, particularly at the gestations of >35–36 weeks, and birthweights >1.70–1.80 kg which are discussed in this chapter (Jones and Roberton, 1986). With modern standards of antepartum and intrapartum care, the intrauterine death of a growth retarded fetus is the exception, as is intrapartum stillbirth or the birth of a severely asphyxiated SFD baby. This is true even when intrauterine growth retardation has not been detected antenatally. Postnatally there is an increased incidence (3–6 per cent) of malformation in SFD babies. Many of the malformed babies have major and rapidly fatal disorders like Potter's syndrome or trisomy 13 and often weigh < 1.50 kg at birth; others with, say, congenital heart defects or neural tube defects are only mildly growth retarded, are often above the 10th centile, never mind the 3rd centile, and are treatable. Although it is often said that smallness-for-dates should induce the physician to examine the neonate with greater care to seek out malformations this is an unjustified view. Not only should *all* neonates be carefully examined for malformations, but in any case most of the malformations in SFD babies are howlingly obvious and do not need to be ferreted out. It is not worth screening SFD infants for evidence of congenital infection unless some of the other stigmata of the conditions are present (p. 227–31).

If a serious malformation is detected which is life

threatening, or needs surgery, then that baby needs neonatal unit admission, but for the other 94–99 per cent of small-for-dates babies > 1.7 kg birthweight, PNW care is ideal so long as hypoglycaemia can be prevented.

MEDICAL CARE OF SFD NEONATES

The general management of these small babies, in particular the prevention of early hypothermia to which they are particularly prone, is outlined above (p. 178).

Medical problems purported to be more common in SFD babies include an increased incidence of infection, polycythaemia, coagulation disturbances, hypothermia and meconium aspiration. However, in our experience the first three conditions are not a problem in the general population of SFD babies, nor is meconium aspiration which, contrary to common belief, is more of a hazard of postmaturity than small-ness-for-dates.

In our experience, therefore, the only important medical problem in the live-born, normally formed, SFD baby is hypoglycaemia, and anxiety about that problem is what motivates many physicians, incorrectly I believe, to admit such babies to a neonatal unit with all the attendant disadvantages outlined in Chapter 10. The rest of this section will, therefore, deal in detail with the prevention, detection and, if necessary, the management of hypoglycaemia in SFD babies weighing > 1.70 kg at birth.

HYPOGLYCAEMIA IN SFD NEONATES

Definition
(p. 277)

Small-for-dates babies do not develop symptoms of neuroglycopenia, that is fits or apnoea, unless the blood glucose has been below 1.0 mmol/l for several hours. The present controversy about hypoglycaemia is dealt with in detail on pp. 277–9. In general the management of SFD babies is geared to keeping their blood glucose >1.5–2.0 mmol/l in the first 48–72 hours and responding briskly, but without panic, to levels below this in asymptomatic neonates.

Prevention of hypoglycaemia – feeding

The prevention of hypoglycaemia in SFD infants, rather than its treatment, is the correct approach. Furthermore, in our experience it is a successful approach, since if SFD babies are fed according to the routine (Table 11.1) symptomatic hypoglycaemia can be prevented, and asymptomatic hypoglycaemia made very rare (Jones and Roberton, 1986).

Monitoring for hypoglycaemia

In SFD neonates symptomatic hypoglycaemia only develops after a period of several hours of asymptomatic hypoglycaemia (<1.0 mmol/l) during which brain function is sustained by the metabolism of other fuels such as ketones and lactate (p. 279). In SFD babies and those with Clifford's syndrome, it is entirely safe therefore for blood glucose to be monitored routinely by Dextrostix or BM stix at 2, 6, 12, 18, 24, 36 and 48 hours of age, the 18 hour estimation only being necessary in the smaller and more premature infant. Asymptomatic or symptomatic hypoglycaemia rarely if ever occurs after 48 hours of age in SFD babies who are feeding satisfactorily. Therefore, so long as feeding is going well by 48 hours of age there is no need to monitor blood glucose in bottle-fed babies. However, if there are any anxieties about the adequacy of feeding in a breast-fed, small-for-dates baby his Dextrostix/BM stix should be monitored 8–12 hourly for a further 24–48 hours.

We have found that Dextrostix/BM stix estimations using the Glucometer to read the reagent strip are entirely satisfactory for this purpose, but it is important to confirm Glucometer values < 1.5 mmol/l by doing a true blood glucose estimation in the laboratory since the major inaccuracy of the reagent strips is to *under*-read at low levels of true glucose.

TREATMENT OF HYPOGLYCAEMIA

With the feeding regime outlined below, even asymptomatic hypoglycaemia is very rare. However, if a low Dextrostix/BM stix is found, while the result is being confirmed, the baby is given the next feed due, irrespective of the time since the last feed. The routine for this depends on whether the baby is breast-fed (p. 187) or bottle-fed (p. 189). In most cases, this causes an acceptable rise in the blood glucose and the pre-existing feeding routine should then continue, but the Dextrostix should be checked 3–4 hourly during the next 12 hours. If there is a tendency for the blood glucose to fall to the 1.0–1.5 mmol/l range before the next 3-hourly feed, then it may be necessary to change to 2-hourly tube feeds for 12–24 hours, putting the baby to the breast, if relevant, for alternate feeds.

If the blood glucose does not rise above 1.0 mmol/l with the extra feed, or the baby vomits, or if he is symptomatic (apnoea or fits) he should be admitted to the neonatal unit and 10 ml of 10 per cent dextrose given intravenously at once followed by an intravenous infusion of 10 per cent dextrose at 60–90 ml/kg/24 hours.

FEEDING LOW BIRTHWEIGHT BABIES

The principles of feeding babies between 1.8–2.5 kg whether they are pre-term or small-for-dates is much the same, though as the SFD baby is much more prone to hypoglycaemia, much greater care has to be taken to monitor for this complication. If it is developing, a much more vigorous complementary or supplementary feeding regimen must be instituted in those babies who are breast-fed (see below).

The dangers of symptomatic hypoglycaemia which may cause serious, permanent brain damage are such that they outweigh the theoretical hazards of cows' milk allergy/intolerance, and it is therefore important to give such babies complementary or supplementary feeds of formula.

BREAST-FEEDING

If the mother is intending to breast-feed her SFD or 32–36 week baby he should, as always, go to the breast in the labour ward (pp. 79, 144).

In addition, irrespective of other complications such as hypoglycaemia, she should put her baby to the breast 3 hourly through the next 48 hours so that he obtains the colostrum and stimulates her lactation. The 3-hourly routine is recommended since it is recognised that these babies do better with small frequent feeds, and with the shorter interfeed interval, hypoglycaemia is less likely. In babies at the smaller end of the range, nearer 32–33 weeks' gestation or 1.7–2.0 kg, it is a matter of clinical judgment whether or not to give them complementary feeds by bottle or tube during the first 48–72 hours, or indeed after this time. However, so long as the blood glucose (Dextrostix) stays above 1.5 mmol/l there is probably no need to do this.

If a low blood glucose value is found (p. 185) a feed should be offered straight away and the rise in blood glucose checked by a further measurement immediately after the feed. Unless the baby is breast-feeding very well and the mother's lactation well established, this additional feed should be of formula giving 15–20 ml/kg/feed. If the mother's own EBM is available, this is of course preferable and can be given by bottle or tube. If the blood glucose has not risen more than 0.2–0.5 mmol/l, consideration should be given to admitting the baby to NNICU for i.v. glucose.

If a breast-fed pre-term or SFD baby has started complementary feeds for hypoglycaemia at any time in the first 24–48 hours, complementary feeds should probably be continued throughout the rest of that period, and until the mother's milk comes in. Complements of 60 ml/kg should be given on day one divided in to eight feeds, and 90 ml/kg on day two in eight feeds (Table 11.1).

After the first 48–72 hours, problems with hypoglycaemia are very unusual, particularly in babies who have been previously normoglycaemic and in SFD babies who often feed voraciously. A more relaxed attitude to demand feeding can then be taken, though babies weighing < 2.00 kg normally need to breast-feed at least 3 hourly, and if they are not doing so a careful watch should be kept on the Dextrostix/BM stix and weight gain. However, by the time they have reached 2.30–2.50 kg they are usually naturally stretching out the interfeed interval to 4 hourly.

Breast-feeding problems in small babies are coped with as outlined on p. 153 et. seq., but as might be expected, recourse to tube feeding while the problems are ironed out is much more often necessary. However, this is unusual in the 35–36 weeks baby, or the mature SFD one, but getting the 32–33 weeks baby to suckle successfully demands patience from the mother and skilled nursing support. Demoralisation in all parties (nurse, mother, paediatrician and baby) is not uncommon, and tube feeding may be necessary. It is rare, however, for healthy well grown babies over 33 weeks GA to require more than 3–4 days of complete tube feeding, plus a further 7–10 days when some tube feeding feeds are needed, after which the mother feels the glow of achievement as her 1.80 kg baby thrives at the breast.

Although 1.70–2.00 kg babies are less likely to achieve satisfactory breast-feeding than full term ones, I believe that one of the great advantages of caring for these babies on a postnatal ward is that satisfactory breast-feeding is more likely to be achieved than if the mother and baby are separated by admitting the baby to a NNICU. The figure of 55 per cent for breast-feeding on discharge in such babies is, we believe, very satisfactory (Whitby *et al.*, 1982).

BOTTLE-FEEDING

Inevitably, managing feeding in pre-term and SFD babies is easier if the mother chooses to bottle-feed rather than breast-feed.

Bottle-fed babies < 2.50 kg should also be demand fed, but aiming for a 3-hourly schedule or eight feeds per day, changing towards a 4-hourly schedule and six feeds per day by the time they are 2.50 kg. The babies should probably be offered one of the standard neonatal formulae (Table 9.3) progressing after a few days to one of the newer pre-term follow-on formulae (Table 9.5) in the volumes given in Table 11.1. If most of this is taken, and the baby is not becoming hypoglycaemic, nothing more needs to be done. One of the great advantages of bottle-feeding is, of course, that one knows exactly how much milk a baby is taking, and if he is not taking enough, and in particular if there are problems with his weight, hypoglycaemia or jaundice, he should be topped up down a tube.

TABLE 11.1 Volumes of milk to feed to normal 1.80–2.50 kg pre-term and SFD neonates

Day	Volume/kg/24 hours
1	60
2	90
3	120
4	150
7–10	180–200

Other feeding problems are dealt with as outlined in Chapter 9.

TUBE FEEDING

Indication

The decision to use tube feeds is usually based on several factors including:

- The number of times a baby wakes for a feed – too often or too few.
- How well he suckles during the feed.
- How much milk he ultimately takes despite apparent initial hunger and enthusiasm.
- The amount of weight lost, or the paucity of weight gain.
- Dextrostix/BM stix readings.

Probably the most common indication for tube feeding is the small-for-dates baby within the first 24–48 hours whose Dextrostix is hovering around the 1.0 mmol/l level and in whom a true glucose estimation comes back at, say, 0.8 mmol/l. This baby should immediately be fed, and as he is often unenthusiastic about it, this should be given down the tube. Another clear indication for a tube-feed is a 6-day-old baby, breast- or bottle-fed, who has lost 8–10 per cent of his birthweight and his Dextrostix is only 1.0–1.5 mmol/l.

Less dramatically, if a baby is bottle-fed, is falling 20–30 per cent short of the desired intake per day (Table 11.1), and his weight gain is poor, some tube feeds should be given. With breast-feeding infants, since test weighing should initially be avoided (p. 153), the only guide is the blood glucose, the weight gained and feeding enthusiasm, and if these are substandard, tube feeding should again be considered. In many such babies, all that is usually required is one or two supplementary or complementary tube feeds before they settle in to a satisfactory feeding pattern. In babies at 32–33 weeks gestational age whose attempts at breast- or bottle-feeding are clearly hopeless, however, a routine of full tube feeding should be instituted.

Management of tube feeds

These can be given very successfully by the mother (after instruction) on a postnatal ward and logistically it is easier to organise if the baby is bottle-fed; he merely gets the necessary volume of milk down his tube every 3 (or 4) hours.

If he is breast-fed, in general he should be given the chance of going to the breast first, both to stimulate his mother's lactation and also to boost her morale. He should then receive a complementary tube feed of appropriate volume (see above). However, if he is clearly hopeless at fixing and suckling, full tube feeding should be instituted, attempting every 48–72 hours to re-interest him in fixing at the breast.

Commonly, an intermediate situation applies; the baby feeds well sometimes, or to start with, but does not consistently take enough milk, gain weight, or keep his blood glucose satisfactory. Conventional wisdom in this situation is that the baby should be given alternate tube and bottle/breast-feeds, rather than have each breast- or bottle-feed topped up by a complementary tube feed.

The decision to graduate from all tube feeds to alternate tube and bottle/breast-feeds, and then to full normal feeding is a clinical one based on assessment of the baby's general condition, alertness, enthusiasm for trial feeds and weight gain.

Throughout the period of tube feeding, the mother should try to keep her lactation going by regularly emptying her breasts either by manual expression or by using a breast pump (p. 152). The milk produced can then be given down the tube to her baby.

If she is not producing enough milk, standard infant formula should be given down the nasogastric tube, progressing to the pre-term follow-on formulae once the baby starts to nipple-feed satisfactorily.

Technique

Nasogastric or orogastric tubes should be used and each have their protagonists. Oral tubes are marginally easier to pass, and do not have the disadvantage that they partially obstruct the nasal airways. However, they cannot be left in situ, and if more than an occasional tube feed is likely to be necessary, I believe an indwelling 4-FG nasogastric feeding tube should be inserted. It is perfectly possible to breast- or bottle-feed with an indwelling NG tube, and the baby is spared the unpleasantness of repeated tube passage. The position of the tube should be confirmed by aspirating acid gastric contents or by auscultation over the stomach while blowing 5 ml of gas down the tube. The tube must be firmly anchored at the nose, and should be aspirated before the start of each feed. This is not only essential to confirm that the tube is still in the stomach, but identifies those babies who are not tolerating oral feeding and have milk pooling in their stomachs; such babies often need neonatal unit admission for further evaluation and treatment.

To give the tube feed, the appropriate volume of milk should be allowed, under the influence of gravity, to run down in to the stomach from some receptacle; a 20 ml syringe is very useful. It should never be syringed in, other than to overcome the surface tension of bubbles in the tube at the start of a feed. The milk should flow in freely usually over a period of 5–20 minutes depending on the volume.

Volume and frequency

In general, pre-term and SFD babies need 3-hourly tube feeds, and the volume given (based on Table 11.1) should be divided into a 3-hourly feeding schedule. Within our PNW routine we are prepared to give 2-hourly tube feeds for a day or two, but usually babies who need them this frequently, and all babies needing hourly tube feeds are transferred to the neonatal unit.

If the tube feed is complementing a bottle-feed, the deficit should be made up. If the tube feed is being given following a breast-feed in the first few days when only colostrum is likely to have been taken, the full volume should be given (Table 11.1). Thereafter, a smaller proportion can be given based on clinical assessment, the Dextrostix, the weight gain and hydration of the baby, and the result of any previous test weighing. If alternate tube- and breast- or bottle-feeds are being given the appropriate volume due at that 3-hourly feed should be given by tube.

DISCHARGING SMALL BABIES

Both breast-fed and artificially fed pre-term and SFD babies can be discharged once they are feeding and gaining weight satisfactorily, and can maintain their body temperature in a 21°C postnatal ward. Some assessment of the parents and their home circumstances should be made to ensure that they understand the feeding regimes necessary in a 1.80–2.00 kg baby, and also understand the implications of, and have the wherewithal to keep the baby adequately clothed and his bedroom at 21°C. Particularly if the baby's weight is still below 2.00 kg collaboration with the district midwife, health visitor and general practitioner should be assured so that the baby is adequately supervised once discharged. In general the mature but SFD baby is ready for discharge sooner than the pre-term one.

POST-DISCHARGE CARE

MILK FEEDS

In view of the data on better weight gain using the specially fortified formulae for ex-prems these milks should in general be recommended for use after discharge (Table 9.5).

VITAMINS

Pre-term babies should be given iron (60 mg o.d. $FeSO_4$) and vitamin supplement (Abidec 0.6 ml o.d.) until they are 6 months old, since they have missed out on some of the maternal-fetal transfer of these substances which occurs primarily in the third trimester. However, this is probably not necessary for SDF babies unless prolonged exclusive breast-feeding is intended.

MILESTONES

The parents should be warned that babies achieve their milestones at a given time from conception. A baby born 7 weeks prematurely will therefore probably not smile until he is 13–15 weeks old rather than at 8 weeks, which is what the parents may be expecting.

IMMUNISATIONS

The standard triple, Hib and polio immunisation should be given according to the baby's chronological age. No allowance should be made for his prematurity, which is emphatically *not* a contraindication for the pertussis component of the vaccine.

REFERENCES

Hey, E.N. (1971). The care of babies in incubators. In: *Recent Advances in Paediatrics*. Eds. D.T.M. Gairdner and D. Hull. J. & A. Churchill, London, pp. 171–216.

Jones, R.A.K. and Roberton, N.R.C. (1986). Small-for-dates babies, are they really a problem? *Archives of Disease in Childhood* **61**, 877–880.

Whitby, C., deCates, C.R. and Roberton, N.R.C. (1982). Infants weighing 1.8–2.50 kg: should they be cared for in a neonatal unit or postnatal ward? *Lancet* **i**, 322–325.

12

TWINS

TYPES OF TWIN

There are two types of twin, monozygous and dizygous. Monozygous or identical twins arise from the division of a single fertilised zygote early in embryogenesis. This type of twinning has a very consistent incidence in all communities and races of about 3–4/1000 pregnancies, and this condition does not, in general, show a familial tendency.

Dizygous or non-identical twins arise from two ova being simultaneously fertilised and implanting together. This type of twinning tends to run in families, and is responsible for the different incidence of twinning in different races which varies from about 1/1000 in Japan to 50/1000 in Nigeria. Dizygous twinning is also a feature of increasing maternal age.

ESTABLISHING ZYGOSITY

In the neonatal period monozygosity can be assumed if there is a monochorial placenta (Fig. 12.1), or with the very rare monoamniotic placentation. In a monoamniotic placenta the twins share a single amniotic cavity. Serious congenital malformations are common in this rare situation. In monochorionic placentae the two amniotic cavities are separated by amnioin only (Fig. 12.1) and this is clearly evident when attempting to separate the two sacs after delivery of the placenta. It is also easily recognised histologically. A dichorioinic placenta can also occur in monozygous twins. Examination of the placenta and

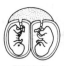 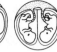

Dichorionic Diamniotic	Dichorionic Diamniotic	Monochorionic Diamniotic	Monochorionic Monoamniotic
Di – or Mono-zygous		Monozygous	Monozygous

FIGURE 12.1 Types of twinning showing variation in membranes and placentae.

fetal membranes, which should always be done in twin pregnancies, can therefore confirm monozygosity (i.e. monoamniotic, or monochorial placenta). However, it cannot exclude monozygosity (or confirm dizygosity), since a dichorioinic placenta occurs in both types of twins. Twins of different sex are clearly dizygous. The only difficulty, therefore, occurs in like-sexed twins with a dichorionic placenta. Some of these clearly look different even in the neonatal period, e.g. hair colour, ear shape, facial contours, but if assessing zygosity is important, blood grouping and HLA typing will usually make the answer clear.

MEDICAL CARE OF TWINS

Since historic times, and in many primitive communities to this day, twins have been regarded as an ill omen, and twins still have a higher perinatal mortality and neonatal mortality due to the markedly increased incidence of pre-term labour in twin pregnancy, and the higher incidence of malformations in twins. However, once the mother with twins has got to 32–33 weeks gestation, the babies have been delivered in good condition, and have no signs of any neonatal illness including things specific to twins, like twin–twin transfusion syndrome, then they have no more problems than singleton babies of the same weight and gestation. Nevertheless, twins are frequently and unnecessarily admitted to the NNICU, and twinning is still listed as a (presumably acceptable) cause of death by the Office of Population Censuses and Surveys.

Striking differences in birthweight may occur. This may be even more than 1.0 kg, and is particularly common in the presence of the twin–twin transfusion syndrome (see below). Differences in birthweight and the presence of disease in just one of a twin pair raises the problem of whether twins should always be kept together after delivery. As a general rule, I believe that they should – even if this means some bending of the rules outlined in Chapter 10 – e.g. putting a 1.60 kg baby on a PNW to be with his 2.20 kg sibling, or keeping the healthy asymptomatic 2.20 kg twin on the NNICU to be with his ill sibling. However, if it is clear that one is going to need prolonged NNICU care, and the other does not, I would let the mother have them one at a time, recognising the risk that the one she gets could well become her 'favourite'.

The medical management of twins is, however, no different from that outlined in Chapter 11 for normal, singleton, pre-term, or SFD babies. However, there are a few problems specific to the management of twins, and feeding two babies clearly poses problems.

CONGENITAL MALFORMATIONS

The incidence of malformation is high in twin pregnancy, indeed monozygous twinning could be regarded as a malformation. However, so long as a twin has a normal clinical examination after birth, this anxiety should not influence his subsequent management.

TWIN–TWIN TRANFUSION SYNDROME

Monozygous monochorionic twins may share vascular channels within the placenta. Where channels are shared, a balanced circulatory pattern may occur, but more commonly the result is that one twin tends to bleed into the other twin so that one becomes very plethoric (the recipient) and the other very anaemic (the donor). In general the donor twin is smaller than the recipient, and may even die. The donor to go in to heart failure and become plethoric and even hydropic. Differences in haemoglobin of 5 g/l or less are unlikely to cause problems unless the lower twin is < 10 g/l. With bigger haemoglobin differences, there will be the problems of anaemia and polycythaemia respectively and NNICU admission is often necessary.

SMALL-FOR-DATES TWINS

It must be emphasised that no concessions can be made in assessing smallness-for-dates just because of multiple pregnancy. If a baby is less than the 3rd centile, irrespective of whether he is a twin, triplet or a sextuplet, he is small-for-dates, and must be managed as such. Twins, therefore, commonly have to be managed as SFD neonates. Indeed there is some evidence to suggest that the SFD second twin is particularly at risk from hypoglycaemia.

FEEDING

If the mother is going to bottle-feed, there are no specific problems other than those described for premature or SFD babies in Chapter 11. The problems come if she wants to breast-feed, which indeed she should be encouraged to do. Given that the average healthy woman produces about 800 ml, or at the outside 1000 ml of milk a day, this means that there is only 400–500 ml/baby per day, which in turn means that if a baby needs 150–170 ml/kg/day, twins can only usually be exclusively breast-fed until they are at maximum 3.50 kg each. There is also the problem that if they are to be exclusively breast-fed only one person can do it!

There are various feeding alternatives for the mother of twins:

1 Feed both twins simultaneously, one at each breast.

2 Feed them sequentially, one at each breast.

3 As above, adding a complementary feed of 50–60 ml of formula at some feeds if weight gain has been poor. Or give one or two full bottle-feeds a day, giving all the rest as breast-feeds.

4 Express one breast and let the father feed one twin with the EBM in a bottle, while the other twin suckles at the other breast; alternate which twin has the privilege of the breast-feed.

5 At a given feed put one twin to the breast, and give the other one a bottle, again alternating the one which has the privilege of the breast-feed.

6 Give one twin all breast-feeds and the other all bottle-feeds.

7 Bottle-feed both.

Apart from the last alternative, all these have problems of potentially poor weight gain in the baby, inconvenience for the mother, confusion for the baby if he is offered a choice of nipples to suck on, and conflict of feelings if one twin gets more 'breast' than the other. In general, however, I would recommend starting with the first two techniques and then go to the fifth when the milk supply cannot meet the demand. Whichever routine is used, however, it is particularly important to document the baby's weight gain to ensure that the 30 g/day average is being sustained (p. 83). If this is not happening, the usual cause is an inadequate intake, and appropriate complementary or supplementary feeds should be given (see p. 186 et. seq.).

DISCHARGING TWINS

The usual criteria for discharge have to be met: the babies are feeding, thriving, and staying warm, and the home environment has been checked and is satisfactory. As with admitting twins, the attempt should always be made to keep them together despite the apparent appeal of discharging one home first and letting the mother get used to one new baby, before she has to get used to two. However, if it is clear that several weeks are going to elapse between the first and second twin going home, separation should be allowed. Like all family members, the twin at home should be encouraged to visit regularly, to see his sibling still in the hospital.

WELL BABY CARE

VITAMINS, IMMUNISATION, MILESTONES, CHOICE OF FORMULA

The management of these is no different from those affecting singletons (p. 194).

Non-identical twins are likely to be as different as any pair of siblings, and their growth and development may differ accordingly. If there was marked discordance in their birthweight, even though they may be identical, the smaller one is always likely to stay smaller.

TRIPLETS AND HIGHER MULTIPLES

With increasing use of ovulation-stimulating drugs and in vitro fertilisation the number of triplets and higher multiples delivered is increasing. Because of the total size of the conceptus (all the babies plus all the placentae) in triplet and higher multiple pregnancies, pre-term labour is almost inevitable.

However, some women, with triplet pregnancies in particular, may manage to get through to 33–35 weeks gestation before they go into pre-term labour.

The management of all three babies is then exactly the same as that for twins or indeed that of singletons. So long as they are asymptomatic and above 1.70–1.80 kg, they can be perfectly satisfactorily managed on a postnatal ward with their mother. Indeed the sooner the poor woman learns the problems of coping with three babies the better, though quite clearly the staff on a postnatal ward would have to give her considerable help in organising the feeding and changing three babies in the first few days.

For obvious reasons, breast-feeding triplets poses a major problem, though there is no reason at all why the mother should not sustain her lactation and give her babies occasional doses of breast milk – for example feeding one of the three at each breast feed.

FURTHER READING

Bryan, E.M. (1992). *Twins and Higher Multiple Births*. Edward Arnold, London, Melbourne, Auckland.

13

BIG BABIES

INTRODUCTION

Most babies who weigh more than the 97th centile for their gestational age (Table 13.1) are entirely normal but large babies, often with large and equally normal parents. However, being large at birth may be a result of fetal illness or malformation, or maternal illness, in particular diabetes (Table 13.2). It has been suggested that the large-for-dates baby whose birthweight is >97th centile merits as close scrutiny as the SFD baby, and there is no doubt at all that large babies do have an increased perinatal morbidity and mortality primarily due to the sequelae of the physical problems of getting out of a conventionally sized birth canal (Table 13.3). Their perinatal mortality is roughly double that of normally grown term babies, and if they weigh >5.00 kg at birth their perinatal mortality may be 10 times higher.

TABLE 13.1 97th centile for males and females at different gestations (Yudkin *et al.*, 1987)

GA (wk)	Males (kg)	Females (kg)
34	3.08	3.00
35	3.37	3.26
36	3.64	3.50
37	3.88	3.71
38	4.09	3.89
39	4.25	4.05
40	4.36	4.16
41	4.40	4.24
42	4.39	4.25

TABLE 13.2   Causes of large babies

- Maternal diabetes
- Heavy/large mothers
- Postmaturity
- Hydrops/ascites
- Transposition of great vessels
- Rare syndromes
  Beckwith-Wiedemann
  Sotos
  Marshall
  Weaver

Since largeness-for-dates is a marker of maternal diabetes, some obstetricians would regard the birth of such a baby as an indication for checking the mother for diabetes either in the puerperium or in her next pregnancy.

From the point of view of the large baby however, if he escapes the intrapartum problems (Table 13.3) and is delivered undamaged and unasphyxiated, he poses few problems in the neonatal period. Four points, nevertheless, are worth noting: feeding, weight, jaundice and weaning.

TABLE 13.3   Morbidity in large-for-dates neonates

Birth asphyxia

- Low Apgar score
- Meconium aspiration
- Hypoxic-ischaemic encephalopathy
- Shoulder dystocia

Birth trauma

- Fractures:
  Clavicle and long bones
- Brachial plexus palsy (Erb's)
- Subdural haemorrhage
- Bruising, cephalhaematomata etc.

FEEDING

A 5.00 kg baby needs 750–800 ml milk/day. This is getting close to the average production during established lactation of the normal woman who was designed to produce enough milk to provide for a 3.50 kg baby for 4–6 months.

It is, therefore, going to be very difficult for most women to sustain adequate growth and weight gain in their exclusively breast-fed 5 kg birthweight hulk for more than 2–3 months at the outside.

WEIGHT

Normal babies may lose up to 10 per cent of their body weight in the neonatal period. In a 5.00 kg baby this means 500 g, i.e. more than 1 lb, and this can alarm both the mother and nursing staff. Furthermore, because of the enormous caloric demands of such a large baby compared with his mother's capacity for milk production in the first 4–5 days he is more likely to lose a lot of weight than a 3.50 kg baby whose fluid and caloric requirements are more easily met by breast-feeding. However, so long as the big baby is otherwise well, sucks and feeds well, and the mother's milk has come in, there is every reason to persevere with just breast-feeding so long as the baby starts to gain weight by the fourth or fifth day at the approved 30 g/day. In general during the first few months babies born >97th centile tend to drift towards the 50–75th centile for all measurements. This is not failure to thrive, it is normal.

JAUNDICE

Big babies are more likely to become jaundiced in the neonatal period because of:
• poor fluid intake per kilogram body weight,

particularly if breast-fed (see above);
- increased risk of trauma bruising/cephal-haematomata during delivery (p. 238).

However, the management of jaundice in such babies is no different from that outlined in Chapter 17.

WEANING

Because of their large caloric requirements, and often voracious appetite, the question is often raised whether these infants should be weaned earlier than the 4–6 months recommended for conventionally sized babies. In general the answer is yes, though perhaps weaning foods should be offered no earlier than three months. Ideally, as hypoallergenic a food as possible, such as rice cereals should be used; delay gluten (wheat) based cereals for as long as possible (p. 22).

REFERENCE

Yudkin, P.L., Aboualfa, M., Eyre, J.A., Redman, C.W.G. and Wilkinson, A.R. (1987). New birthweight and head circumference centiles for gestational age 24–42 weeks. *Early Human Development* 15, 45–52.

FURTHER READING

Stevenson, D.K., Hopper, A.O., Cohen, R.S., Bucalo, L.R., Kerner, J.A. and Sunshine, P. (1982). Macrosomia: causes and consequences. *Journal of Pediatrics* 100, 515–520.

14

POSTMATURE BABIES

—

By definition these are babies born at 294 days of gestation or more. The main purpose in giving them a separate chapter is to emphasise three points:

- Postmaturity is a problem for obstetricians since prolonged pregnancy increases the risk of fetal death and intrapartum stillbirth. Intrapartum asphyxia, and in particular meconium aspiration pneumonia, is also more common with postmature pregnancies. However, if these problems develop they are obvious at birth and the neonate needs neonatal unit admission.

- Postmaturity is *not* the same as smallness-for-dates, though clearly a baby can be both in which case he should be managed as outlined in Chapter 11. In particular postmature normal birthweight babies are not prone to hypoglycaemia unless they fulfil the diagnostic criteria of Clifford's syndrome (p. 182).

- *Most important:* if postmature babies escape the above hazards they are normal babies and should be treated as such on the PNW.

POSTNATAL WARD CARE

Because these babies are mature they feed well, have livers that conjugate bilirubin well, rarely become ill and do not require special attention on a PNW. They have dry and wrinkled skin and long finger nails with which they scratch themselves.

The skin does not need treatment, and the nails can either be clipped or the baby can wear mittens.

15

THE INFANT OF THE DIABETIC MOTHER

INTRODUCTION

In the last 10–15 years the quality of control imposed on pregnant diabetic women has improved out of all recognition. This has had three major effects:

- The perinatal mortality of infants of diabetic mothers (IDM) has fallen to very low levels; only malformations and the outcome of pregnancies in uncooperative patients keep the PNM marginally higher than that seen in non-diabetics.
- The gestation at which diabetic mothers are delivered has increased from an average of 36–37 weeks to 39–40 weeks.
- The typical rotund large-for-dates (>97th centile) IDM is now rarely seen.

As a result, I believe it is now entirely safe to transfer a mature IDM who is asymptomatic in the labour ward to the PNW with his mother. This applies to infants of long-term diabetics who have been on insulin for years, to infants of gestational diabetics who were given insulin only during pregnancy, and also to infants of gestational diabetics who required only dietary control in pregnancy. Should the obstetrician have been unwise enough to give oral hypoglycaemic drugs to the mother in pregnancy (p. 47) prolonged and profound neonatal hypoglycaemia can be anticipated, and any such neonate should be admitted to the neonatal unit.

HYPOGLYCAEMIA

For the normally formed IDM with no early onset respiratory disease, the major anxiety is hypoglycaemia.

PATHOPHYSIOLOGY OF HYPOGLYCAEMIA IN IDM

Throughout pregnancy the fetal blood glucose is in equilibrium with the maternal levels. In an infant of a poorly controlled diabetic mother the fetal blood glucose value will also have been high, stimulating the fetal islets of Langerhans. As a result, the fetus will be hyperinsulinaemic, and is likely to stay hyperinsulinaemic after delivery, when, in the absence of the transplacental supply of glucose, the high insulin levels will cause marked early onset hypoglycaemia (Fig. 15.1), often reaching a nadir around 1.0 mmol/l by 1–2 hours of age. However, as Fig. 15.1 also shows, the normal trend is for the glucose in such infants to rise spontaneously by 3–4 hours of age. With good maternal control, many IDM do not drop their blood glucose into the hypoglycaemic range, though they all show a rapid postnatal fall in glucose levels. Despite this rapid metabolic change in the first 2–3 hours, the infants rarely show symptoms, though they are often slightly quieter than usual and may be a little pale and sweaty; fits and apnoea do not occur. There is no evidence that this transient hypoglycaemia in IDM causes any sequelae whatsoever, and it is for this reason that they can be cared for on a PNW.

TREATMENT

Two things are important:
- To ensure that if the blood glucose falls to 1.0 mmol/l it rises again by 4 hours.
- To minimise the incidence of such hypoglycaemia by early feeding.

The blood glucose should be measured by Dextrostix

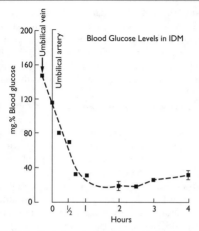

FIGURE 15.1 Blood glucose levels in infants with diabetic mothers during the first four hours of life (from Cornblath and Schwartz, 1976, with permission). (40 mg% ≡ 2.2 mmol/l)

or BM stix on admission to the PNW and at 2, 4, 6, and 12 hours of age. The likely response is that the 2 hour level will be low but not necessarily below 1.0 mmol/l. By 4 hours it will be rising from the 2 hour low level up to 1.5–2.0 mmol/l or above, and will stay up thereafter.

The IDM, if otherwise asymptomatic on the PNW, should be fed at 2 hours of age and then 3–4 hourly for the next 12–24 hours. If the mother is intending to bottle-feed, the baby should be given one of the standard infant formulae at the rate of 60 ml/kg/24 hours by tube if necessary.

If the mother is intending to breast-feed, she should suckle the baby at the times of the feeds, but she should in addition complement him with formula as outlined above, unless the Dextrostix or BM stix is staying > 1.50 mmol/l.

After 12–18 hours of age, complements are rarely

required in the breast-fed infant who can then be left to his own devices, and there are no contraindications to a diabetic mother breast-feeding her baby. She will, of course, need to take extra calories and carbohydrate above her normal requirements to sustain her lactation (p. 135), and to cover them with extra insulin.

If the glucose has not risen above 1–1.5 mmol/l by 4 hours (a very unusual event), it may be necessary to give 2-hourly tube feeds for the next 6–12 hours but having to recourse to intravenous dextrose should be regarded as a failure of prenatal, intrapartum and postnatal care.

Infants of diabetic mothers who are on the NNICU because they have respiratory disease, or the aftermath of intrapartum asphyxia, may however pose problems with glucose homeostasis.

OTHER MEDICAL PROBLEMS OF THE IDM

A large number of problems have been described in IDM. However, with the vast improvement in the control of the maternal diabetes alluded to above, these complications are now uncommon. Nevertheless, for reasons that cannot be explained, and despite meticulous control, they may still occasionally develop.

CHARACTERISTIC APPEARANCE AND LARGENESS-FOR-DATES

This is due to the IDM in utero producing an excess of various hormones, including insulin, which stimulate growth. The large baby which results may be damaged during delivery (Chapter 11).

RESPIRATORY DIFFICULTIES

Both RDS and TTN are more common in IDM than normals; with better diabetic control, delivery being delayed until 39–40 weeks, and caesarean section being much less widely used, these complications are now rare.

POLYCYTHAEMIA

IDM tend to have a higher packed cell volume than normals, and this predisposes them to neonatal jaundice. However, I believe polycythaemia is an overused diagnosis (p. 277) and problems attributed to it should only be entertained, and even then not necessarily accepted, if the PCV is > 70 per cent on a central venous sample (not a capillary one which tends to give a falsely high reading).

WEIGHT LOSS

Infants of diabetic mothers often lose close to 10 per cent of their birthweight but so long as no other problems such as jaundice are present, this should not be a cause for concern.

CONGENITAL MALFORMATIONS

Infants of diabetic mothers have an increased incidence of many types of congenital malformations, which are probably related to the quality of periconceptional diabetic control. Congenital heart disease is the most common malformation and includes a specific type of cardiomyopathy with hypertophy of the intraventricular septum leading to heart failure in the neonatal period. The rare malformation of sacral agenesis is also much more common in IDM.

METABOLIC PROBLEMS

Jaundice (Chapter 17), hypocalcaemia (p. 280) and hypomagnesaemia are more common in IDM but rarely cause problems or symptoms which cannot be coped with on a PNW, and their management is no different from that outlined for normal infants in Chapters 17 and 18.

SMALL-FOR-DATES

About 5 per cent of infants of diabetic mothers are small-for-dates. This is usually a marker of severe diabetic vascular disease in the mother. However, the baby, once born, behaves like a typical small-for-dates baby (Chapter 11) and should be managed as such.

POST-DISCHARGE CARE

There are no special features about the post-discharge care of these babies, other than to point out that transient asymptomatic hypoglycaemia is *not* a contraindication to the pertussis component of the triple vaccine.

REFERENCE

Cornblath, M. and Schwartz, R. (1976) *Disorders of carbohydrate metabolism in infancy.* W.B. Saunders Co., Philadephia, London.

FURTHER READING

Cordero, L. and Landon, M.B. (1993). Infant of the diabetic mother. *Clinics in Perinatology* **20**, 635–648.

INFECTION

—

SUSCEPTIBILITY TO INFECTION

The body defends itself against infection in three ways – physical, cellular and humoral. Even full term babies are deficient in all three.

PHYSICAL DEFENCES

The neonatal skin is very thin, easily damaged and infected. The umbilical stump becomes necrotic after birth and acts as a locus for infections which can then disseminate (pp. 75–6). The passage of an endotracheal tube, a nasogastric tube or an intravascular catheter provides a route for pathogenic organisms to enter the body.

The newborn infant is virtually germ-free at birth, apart from organisms smeared over him as he passes through the vagina. He therefore lacks the protection afforded by having a resident flora of non-pathogenic organisms. A normal neonate is colonised by generally non-pathogenic organisms acquired from his mother, including those in her vagina and rectum to which he was exposed during delivery plus those acquired from her skin and upper airway after birth.

CELLULAR IMMUNITY

Lymphocyte function is well developed at term. The absolute number of T cells present is similar to adult values. T cell function seems to be adequate with some decrease in cytotoxic T cell function and in the ability to respond to sensitising agents such as dinitrochlorobenzene.

A full complement of B lymphocyte types is present, and these cells can respond by synthesising antibodies. A swift antibody synthetic response by the neonatal lymphocyte is dependent on there being some IgG in the plasma to help process the antigen. The response of the neonate will, therefore, be improved if he has an adequate level of transplacental maternal IgG.

Polymorphonuclear leucocytes from healthy full term infants when suspended in normal adult serum show normal phagocytosis and bactericidal activity, but some reduction in chemotaxis and adherence. However, when suspended in neonatal serum, deficient in the opsonic activities of immunoglobulins and complement, their phagocytic activity is seriously reduced. The bactericidal capacity of neonatal polymorphs in vivo is also reduced in the presence of severe concurrent illness such as RDS or meconium aspiration pneumonitis.

HUMORAL IMMUNITY

The normal term neonate has no circulating IgA or IgM. IgG is both actively and passively transported across the placenta from about the twentieth week of gestation, and by full term the baby's IgG level is higher than his mother's. Following delivery, the level of the IgG in the infant's plasma falls with a half life of about three weeks, and, until he produces adequate amounts of IgG, IgM and IgA, there is a transient postnatal hypogammaglobulinaemia. This is rarely clinically important in term infants, but premature infants born before much IgG has crossed the placenta have an increased risk of infection from the time of birth for several weeks until after the postnatal hypogammaglobulinaemia has been corrected.

At the trough, about 3–4 weeks after delivery, he may have IgG levels less than 0.2 g/l.

Since the neonate acquires his IgG from his mother, he is immune to the infections to which she is immune, except for those conditions in which immunity is IgM mediated or cell mediated (*E. coli*, TB).

The levels of the components of the complement cascade, and the alternative complement pathway in the neonate, are 50–80 per cent of adult values.

The neonate is immunodeficient because he lacks these defence mechanisms but it is important to recognise that he is immunocompetent since he can, and does, respond to the antigenic challenges he receives postnatally, particularly if he has adequate levels of IgG.

CROSS INFECTION

After delivery, all babies become colonised with bacteria, acquiring organisms on their skin and in their upper and lower airway, mouth and gut. The ideal is that they are colonised with the organisms acquired from their mother (v.s.). It is preferable that he is colonised with these 'community' microbes rather than with the antibiotic resistant, often Gram negative organisms with which hospital staff – nurses and doctors – are colonised. Therefore, his mother should only observe the social graces of cleanliness while handling her newborn baby, though if she has an infectious disease the precautions outlined on pp. 25–8 should apply.

Siblings or other family members with an overt contagious disease should stay away from the new baby both on the PNW and once he is home, and indeed as a general rule should keep away from any other newborn infant. However, the reality is that as soon as most babies go home everyone picks them up and kisses them without any precautions, nor it must be admitted with many apparent ill effects.

The main infectious hazard to the hospitalised neonate is staff, not only because they may be the vectors of baby-to-baby, or infected mother-to-baby, transmission of pathogenic organisms, but primarily because they may transmit to the baby organisms on their own hands, derived from their hair, nose and anywhere else on their body colonised as it is with hospital organisms.

The key to prevention of cross infection is therefore for the staff to be meticulous with their hand washing using an antiseptic soap before and after every occasion they handle a neonate. Chlorhexidine or Betadine soap should be used, not Knight's Castile or Camay, no matter how excellent the latter may be in a domestic setting! Watches and hand jewellery are heavily colonised with pathogenic organisms and should be removed before hand washing (wedding rings are probably just tolerable – but try swabbing under yours and see what grows), and sleeves should be rolled up to the elbow prior to hand washing.

Gowns, masks and overshoes are not required on a routine basis, though if a nurse or a doctor wants to pick up a baby and cuddle him, they should gown, not only to protect the baby from microbes on their clothes, but also to protect their clothes from effluent of various sorts from the baby, particularly if he is naked. Each baby should have his 'own' gown, kept under his cot or in the cot cupboard.

Sharing equipment or lotions between babies should not occur, and each baby should have his own thermometer and pot of zinc and castor oil ointment to apply to his perineum after each nappy change.

Problems with bottle teats are a thing of the past since the 'ready-to-feed' formula preparations (p. 126) come with disposable teats. If teats are to be reused, reuse should be limited to the same baby and they should be kept in a standard Milton solution (dilution 1:20) between feeds, and thoroughly rinsed under a running tap before use.

An important part of the prevention of cross infection on a PNW is good umbilical cord care (p. 75).

INFECTIONS IN THE NURSING AND MEDICAL STAFF

If a nurse has an acute infectious disease, e.g. a respiratory tract infection, gastroenteritis, a viral exanthem, impetigo or infected eczema, she should not be working with newborn babies. Clearly, people with milder upper respiratory tract infections frequently stay on duty, and were such an infection to be transmitted to a term neonate it would rarely, if ever, be serious. However, staff afflicted with an upper respiratory tract infection should mask and be more than usually fastidious with their hand washing, since apart from anything else the presence of such a viral infection considerably increases the likelihood of them shedding organisms such as staphylococci which they carry in their upper airway.

The problem of herpes remains unresolved. Although disseminated neonatal herpes due to herpes virus type 1 acquired from contact with labial herpes or a herpetic whitlow seems to be very rare, the disease is so devastating that it is better to be overcautious. If, because of staff shortages, it is felt that a nurse with an exposed herpetic sore is needed on duty, she should be restricted to non-neonatal chores, apply acyclovir ointment to the lesion and cover it with a mask, gloves or occlusive dressing.

INFECTIONS FROM THE MOTHER

The majority of these problems are dealt with in Table 3.1 on pp. 25–8, and the approach to the baby of a mother who was pyrexial in labour on p. 32; maternal herpes and group B streptococcal carriage, however, merit special attention.

Maternal herpes

The majority of cases of neonatal herpes occur in babies who were *not* delivered through an overtly infected birth canal. The infection is nevertheless derived from the birth canal, but the mother, although shedding the virus intrapartum, was asymptomatic in pregnancy and may never have had symptoms. Conversely, the vast majority of babies born to mothers with previous genital herpes and who therefore may well be shedding the virus asyptomatically during labour do not develop herpes.

In the presence of genital herpes at term, particularly if it is a primary infection, delivery pre-labour or in early labour may be advisable.

If, however, an infant is delivered through an infected birth canal, it is a matter of judgment whether he should be treated with acyclovir from the moment of birth. In most cases where the mother's infection is mild and recurrent, she will have transmitted some antiherpetic IgG antibodies to her baby, and no treatment is indicated unless the baby's skin was damaged (e.g. by a scalp clip) or if he is very premature (< 32 weeks gestation).

In the presence of severe maternal genital herpes the infant should probably be delivered by caesarean section, particularly if it is thought that this was the mother's primary infection (so that she has little antibody to pass to her neonate); such a baby requires no treatment. If he was born *vaginally* through the heavily infected birth canal, or was exposed to prolonged membrane rupture prior to caesarean section, it is probably justifiable to give him a five day course of intravenous acylovir.

Maternal herpes be it labial, genital or a whitlow is not a reason for separating her from her baby, but the mother should be treated with acyclovir, the lesion covered, and she should have a meticulous hand washing routine before dealing with her baby (p. 219).

Maternal group B streptococcus

There is now a plethora of evidence to show that if a woman's genital tract is colonised with GBS when she goes into labour, the chance of her transmitting the infection to her baby can be effectively eliminated by intrapartum ampicillin (0.5–1.0 g i.v.q4h) given throughout labour. Although the evidence is most impressive in women whose membranes have been ruptured for more than 12 hours and are labouring at less than 37 weeks gestational age (Boyer and Gotoff, 1986), GBS sepsis can also kill full term babies and I believe that intrapartum prophylaxis should be offered at all gestations. How to identify the carrier mother is still the subject of research, but much of the evidence suggests that the majority of women who are carriers at the time of delivery also had GBS in their HVS at 28 weeks gestation.

If an asymptomatic infant is born to a mother known to be carrying GBS in her vagina, but who was not treated with antibiotics intrapartum, until the appropriate prospective randomised control trial is done, I prefer to treat all such infants with penicillin; I give 1/4 of a vial of Triplopen* by a single i.m. injection which will give the baby good penicillin levels for 5–7 days.

PROLONGED RUPTURE OF THE MEMBRANES

Except with group B streptococci and herpes (v.s.), the presence of prolonged rupture of the fetal membranes is of no significance if the infant is asymptomatic at the time of birth, and such infants require no treatment. However, if symptoms of any sort, particularly respiratory, develop in the neonate, they

---

*One vial of Triplopen contains 475 mg of benzathine penicillin, 250 mg procaine penicillin and 300 mg benzyl penicillin.

should be assumed to be due to infection and treated as such until cultures prove to be negative.

MINOR INFECTIONS IN NEONATES WHICH CAN BE TREATED ON THE POSTNATAL WARD

UMBILICUS AND SKIN

The umbilical cord should be sprayed at birth with a broad spectrum antibiotic powder, such as Polybactrin, before the cord clamp is attached (p. 75). If this is done properly, it will be rare to see postnatal infection of the umbilicus. If any is detected, with periumbilical redness and local discharge, a swab should be taken. The infection is usually due to staphylococci or *E. coli*, and responds within 2–3 days to a topical antibiotic spray such as Polybactrin administered 2–3 times per day.

If the umbilical cord has been sprayed properly at birth, serious superficial skin infection will also be rare. However, minor superficial infection is not uncommon particularly in the flexures or periumbilically with the formation of small blisters filled with yellowish opalescent fluid. This infection is usually due to staphylococci, and responds to a 5 days' course of oral flucloxacillin (62.5 mg q.d.s). More serious skin infection is rare, but usually presents with either much larger bullae (bullous impetigo, pemphigus neonatorum) or widespread exfoliation of the infant's skin (toxic epidermal necrolysis). These babies require admission to the neonatal unit.

It is important not to treat as infective the many and common neonatal skin rashes which are benign and non-infective (pp. 280–5).

THRUSH

This is usually a trivial oral or perianal infection. It presents with white plaques on the buccal mucosa and tongue which cannot be wiped off, or as the typcial bright erythematous perianal rash with discrete peripheral lesions looking like the base of thin-roofed blisters. The infection may be set up by 'passive' antibiotic administration in breast milk, and may then spread to the mother's nipple, causing cracks and inhibiting breast-feeding. Thrush responds rapidly to topical application of nystatin, amphotericin or miconazole.

CONJUNCTIVITIS

The diagnosis and management of this are outlined in Table 16.1. In many cases, either no organism is cultured or an organism such as *Streptococcus viridans* or *Staphylococcus epidermidis* of doubtful pathogenicity is grown. Treat these babies symptomatically with saline cleansing of the lids if the discharge is mild, changing to 0.5 per cent chloramphenicol if the discharge is more profuse. In a small number of babies with severe conjunctivitis, the lacrymal sac becomes infected (dacryocystitis). This presents as a tender, reddish purple, indurated swelling on the medial side of the lower lid. Treatment with oral antibiotics is indicated as well as the usual eye drops.

URINARY TRACT INFECTION

This commonly presents with mild symptoms such as vomiting, poor weight gain, persisting anaemia or mild jaundice and can usually be managed in the postnatal ward. Occasionally, all the signs of severe sepsis are present, in which case the baby will need to be admitted to the NNICU.

The diagnosis of this condition is of course dependent on urine analysis, and this may be the only positive finding on investigation, since other features of sepsis (p. 294) are often absent in the term neonate with a UTI. It is vital to understand, however, that urine analysis results based on bag specimens of urine collected from neonates should always be viewed with grave suspicion unless pus cells or bacteria are seen

TABLE 16.1

Organism	Age at presentation	Diagnosis	Treatment
Gonococcus	Day 1 (more now recognised in 1st week)	Maternal history – promiscuity etc. Profuse conjunctival discharge Urgent Gram stain on pus shows Gram-ve intracellular diplococci Culture of swab sent in transport medium	i.v. or i.m. penicillin 75 000^U/kg/24 hrs given b.d. for 7 days Penicillin eye drops hourly for 12 hours then 4 hourly for 7 days Notifiable disease Remember to treat mother and consorts
Staph. aureus *E. coli* *Haemophilus*	3–5 days peak but may be at any time including day 1	Culture swab	If mild: sterile saline cleaning If severe: 0.5% chloramphenicol eye drops for 5 days
Chlamydia trachomatis	5+ days	Venereal disease, therefore similar maternal history to G/C Conventional cultures sterile. Immunofluorescence for chlamydia on pus	Chlortetracycline eye ointment q.d.s + systemic erythromycin (30 mg/kg given b.d.) – for 2 weeks

on immediate microscopic examination of the sample in the ward before it was sent to the laboratory.

If a bag urine is normal, then the infant does not have a urinary tract infection. Bag urines with >50 wbc/mm^3 without bacterial growth, or significant bacterial growth (>10^5 organisms/ml) without pus cells or with <50 wbc/mm^3, should not be treated as a UTI. However, a bag urine with a pure growth of >10^5 organisms/ml, plus >100–200 wbc/mm^3, is adequate proof of urinary tract infection, provided that there was no local infection of the perineum or foreskin when the bag sample was collected.

If any doubt exists about the diagnosis of a UTI, urine must be obtained by suprapubic bladder puncture. Any pure growth in the suprapubic sample, irrespective of the number of organisms present, indicates a UTI.

Whenever a UTI is diagnosed, check whether any antenatal abnormalities had been found by ultrasound of the fetal renal tract, and also examine the infant carefully to exclude renal, bladder or genital abnormalities, and in particular exclude posterior urethral valves in males (pp. 94–5). Measure his BP.

In infants with a few or no symptoms treat with oral antibiotics such as amoxicillin (62.5 mg q.d.s). This can be changed if necessary once sensitivities are available, and treatment should be given for 7–10 days. The more seriously ill infant will need NNICU admission and parenteral antibiotics.

Once a UTI has been diagnosed, the neonate should have his urea and electrolytes checked, and the urinanalysis repeated following completion of therapy. The renal tract must also be investigated. The current fashion is to do a renal ultrasound scan, a DTPA or MAG 3 scan, and a cystogram.

GASTROENTERITIS

Severe nursery epidemics of gastroenteritis due to salmonella, shigella, enteropathogenic *E. coli.* and viruses still occasionally occur. Infection with the rotavirus is endemic in some neonatal units without the infants becoming symptomatic.

Most cases of neonatal gastroenteritis now seen are, however, sporadic and mild, the infants presenting with varying degrees of diarrhoea and vomiting. With prompt recognition of the problem, however, dehydration is rarely seen.

Diagnosis

Stool cultures should be sent from all infants with diarrhoea, though the yield of positive cultures is low.

Treatment

Whenever any neonate develops mild gastorenteritis he should be fed with one of the oral glucose electrolyte solutions such as Dextrolyte. In most cases his symptoms will settle within 24 hours, and he can restart feeding. If the diarrhoea and vomiting does not settle, or dehydration develops, intravenous therapy will be required for 24–48 hours before restarting oral fluids.

Antibiotics should not be given to sporadic cases of neonatal gastroenteritis unless there are clinical signs to suggest that there is systemic spread of the infection. During nursery epidemics due to a bacterial pathogen consider using the oral non-absorbable antibiotics which minimise the amount of cross infection, but may prolong the carrier state.

Isolation

If an infant develops gastroenteritis in the postnatal ward he should not be admitted to the NNICU. If he can be managed with oral treatment, transfer him with his mother to the isolation unit in the maternity hospital, but if the infant requires intravenous therapy he should be transferred to the unit that manages infectious gastroenteritis in older infants.

If it is apparent that an epidemic is under way, depending on the extent of, and organism responsible for, the epidemic, and the severity of illness in the neonates, it may be necessary in consultation with the hospital control of infection committee or team to restrict admissions, close wards, or in extreme cases close the whole maternity unit.

Babies who have recovered from neonatal gastroenteritis but are still shedding pathogens in their stools, can go home if they are feeding and gaining weight well.

Two other points to note about gastroenteritis in the newborn:

- Severe diarrhoea without vomiting which responds to clear fluids, but relapses when milk is reintroduced, suggests congenital lactose (or other sugar) intolerance.
- Many completely asymptomatic infants carry enteropathogenic *E. coli.* (which are usually derived from their mothers) in their stool. No action is required.

SEVERE NEONATAL INFECTION

The recognition of serious neonatal sepsis developing in a neonate on a postnatal ward is described in Chapter 19.

CONGENITAL INFECTIONS

Congenital, i.e. transplacental infection can occur with many organisms (Table 16.2). Many of these organisms only rarely cause truly congenital infection. Those discussed below are of importance in the UK.

CONGENITAL RUBELLA

This is now exceptionally rare in the UK, with fewer than 20 cases per year as a result of generalised childhood immunisation. It does, however, still occur not

TABLE 16.2 Organisms responsible for congenital infection

- Rubella
- Cytomegalovirus
- Toxoplasma
- Herpes
- Varicella
- TB
- Syphilis
- Malaria
- Parvovirus
- HIV
- HTLV I

only in the unimmunised woman, but also in women who have been immunised. In the neonatal period it may present with the extended rubella syndrome, the features of which are listed in Table 16.3, but should also be considered in, for example, babies with just thrombocytopenia or cataract. There is no treatment, but the babies are excreting the virus and should be kept away from women in early pregnancy.

CONGENITAL CYTOMEGALOVIRUS

Congenital CMV may occur following primary infection in the mother, or reactivation of her infection. It is probably the most common congenital infection, affecting up to 1:200 of all births. The majority, including virtually all cases due to reactivation of maternal disease, are asymptomatic in the neonatal period, though some will become deaf on follow-up. A more extended syndrome with many of the features listed in Table 16.3 can occur but it is rare. There is no treatment of proven value. These babies, like those with rubella, shed virus and are an infectious risk to pregnant women and other babies.

CONGENITAL TOXOPLASMOSIS

This is also rare with an incidence in the UK of about 1:10 000 live births. In its most severe form it presents

TABLE 16.3 Features of congenital infection

- Low birthweight for gestational age
- Jaundice
- Hepatosplenomegaly
- Thrombocytopenia: purpura
- Cataract
- Chorioretinitis
- Abnormalities of head growth
  Microcephaly
  Hydrocephalus
  Intracranial calcification
- Osteitis
- Congenital heart disease

with the classic triad of hydrocephalus, intracranial calcification and chorioretinitis. This is, however, very rare and most cases present because the mother was found to have had the disease while pregnant. If the baby is infected, he should be treated with spiramycin (100 mg/kg/day) for 4–6 weeks alternating with pyrimethamine (1 mg/kg/day) plus sulphadiazine (50 mg/kg/day) for 3 weeks, for a whole year.

CONGENITAL SYPHILIS

If overt clinical syphilis is present in the mother, her infant should be fully investigated serologically and have an LP and then be treated with benzyl penicillin (50 000^n/kg) for 10 days. If the significance of a positive maternal serological test for syphilis is uncertain, then the blood of the neonate must be tested for IgM fluorescent treponemal antibody (FTA IgM). If this is positive, it confirms congenital syphilitic infection and the neonate should be treated as outlined above.

CONGENITAL PARVOVIRUS INFECTION

This is the virus of erythema infectiosum (fifth disease) and it also causes aplastic crisis in patients with haemolytic anaemias such as spherocytosis and sickle cell anaemia. Most maternal infections cause no problems, but a small number will abort, and about 1 per cent of their fetuses will develop hydrops.

AIDS

In a sense, this is outside the scope of this book since congenitally infected babies do not present in the neonatal period. However, the disease has several major implications for neonatal practice.

1 In the absence of maternal screening the only safe thing to do is to assume all women and babies are potentially infected. Even if they do not carry HIV, they may carry hepatitis B. Especially in the labour ward gloves should therefore be worn when handling potentially infected material and carrying out procedures in which blood may be spilt. Mouth held mucus extractors must be abandoned.

2 Although in utero transplacental infection can occur, most infection probably occurs around delivery, with approximately 20 per cent of babies of HIV positive mothers ultimately developing AIDS. There is no way of testing a baby in the neonatal period that will identify that 20 per cent. All have antibodies to HIV (maternal-transplacentally acquired). Looking for anti-HIV IgM is not reliable, and techniques to identify the virus in the neonate are also unreliable, though getting better. The diagnosis can only be excluded if, by 15 months of age, the baby is asymptomatic and has undetectable antibody levels.

3 For babies of women known to be infected, hospital guidelines for the management of HIV positive patients must be adhered to. The baby should be nursed with his mother.

4 The infection is probably not a teratogen: there does not seem to be an AIDS phenotype.

5 Breast-feeding by a known infected mother is contraindicated in the developed world.

6 Babies of HIV positive women are at risk from other problems including other sexually transmitted diseases and drug withdrawal syndromes.

7 It is still rare in Britain. Fewer than 200 cases of congenital AIDS had been reported by the end of 1994.

The babies should be fully immunised, including the live MMR vaccine, though the Salk killed polio virus vaccine should be used.

CONGENITAL HTLV INFECTION

This virus, common in patients from Japan or the Caribbean, causes T cell lymphoma and leukaemia in adults. It is transmitted in breast milk. Seropositive women from these communities should therefore be advised not to breast-feed their babies.

REFERENCE

Boyer, K.M. and Gotoff, S.P. (1986). Prevention of early onset neonatal group B streptococcal disease with selective intrapartum chemoprophylaxis. *New England Journal of Medicine* **314**, 1665–1669.

JAUNDICE ON THE POSTNATAL WARD

—

BILIRUBIN PHYSIOLOGY

The haem from 1 g of haemoglobin yields 600 μmol (35 mg) of unconjugated bilirubin, and the normal term infant breaks down about 0.5 g of haemoglobin every 24 hours. Unconjugated bilirubin in the plasma is taken up by the liver where it is combined with two molecules of glucuronic acid by the enzyme glucuronyl transferase to give conjugated bilirubin which enters the bile and passes into the gut. If gut transit time is reduced, conjugated bilirubin is deconjugated by the glucuronidases produced by bacteria in the lumen, and the unconjugated bilirubin is absorbed – the enterohepatic circulation – and once more enters the total pool of unconjugated bilirubin which the liver has to metabolise.

If there is obstruction to bile flow, conjugated bilirubin refluxes from the liver into the plasma and may be excreted in the urine.

KERNICTERUS

Jaundice is an obsession of neonatologists because of the association between raised unconjugated bilirubin levels and permanent neurological sequelae. At postmortem in the neonatal period, a brain damaged this way shows yellow staining of the ganglia of the mid-brain and brain stem – kernicterus – and the clinical syndrome seen in damaged survivors includes various combinations of mental defect, athetoid cerebral palsy and deafness.

The exact mechanism of kernicterus remains unclear. It would appear that in addition to a raised unconjugated bilirubin level something else needs to go wrong. This is most likely to be an insult such as acidaemia, hypoxia or sepsis that disrupts the blood brain barrier, allowing bilirubin to escape from the vascular compartment into the CNS.

Where healthy (apart from being yellow) term babies are concerned, there is no evidence at all that bilirubin levels < 425 μmol/l (25 mg%) are ever associated with CNS sequelae and for similar babies weighing 2.0–2.50 kg the same can be said for bilirubin levels < 300–350 μmol/l (17–20 mg%). These figures need to be very firmly grasped since there is currently a major tendency to panic when bilirubin levels in well babies at home or on a PNW begin to creep into the mid 200 μmol/l range.

PRACTICAL BILIRUBIN CHEMISTRY

In most infants, even those who stay jaundiced for several days, the majority of the bilirubin is present as the unconjugated form, with less than 20–40 μmol/l (1–2 mg%) of conjugated bilirubin. Therefore, the *total* plasma bilirubin – which is what is measured by most of the bilirubinometers in current use in neonatal biochemistry – can be used to measure the total unconjugated bilirubin, and hence the risk of kernicterus.

It is only necessary to measure conjugated bilirubin if the jaundice is prolonged, or if there is other clinical evidence suggesting the presence of obstructive jaundice (Table 17.1).

CLINICAL IMPLICATIONS OF JAUNDICE

If a baby is jaundiced it should alert the clinician to two things:

- Is the level of jaundice so high that kernicterus is a danger?
- Why is the bilirubin high and is it a sign of underlying disease?

To answer the first of these two questions measure the plasma bilirubin. To answer the second question the most important differential feature is the pattern of neonatal jaundice (Fig. 17.1). Each of the four patterns of jaundice shown may be seen in a baby at home or on a PNW.

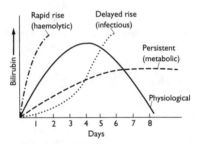

FIGURE 17.1 Pattern of neonatal jaundice (from Roberton, 1993).

RAPID ONSET (DAY 1) JAUNDICE

In these babies the jaundice often appears within the first 12 hours of life, and if serial measurements are made, the bilirubin may be rising faster than 10 μmol/hour.

RHESUS (D) INCOMPATIBILITY

The most important cause of rapid onset jaundice is rhesus (D) incompatibility. Such infants should be identified antenatally as a matter of routine. The more severe cases will often be admitted to the neonatal unit after birth and their management is described by McClure (1992). Many cases of rhesus haemolytic disease of the newborn (HDN) in babies > 36 weeks gestation are, however, mild and after an initial assessment in the NNU and, if neccesary, a first exchange transfusion, are healthy, stable, breast-feeding infants merely at risk from jaundice. They can therefore be cared for on a postnatal ward. They should stay under phototherapy on the postnatal ward until the bilirubin is falling (pp. 243–5). Their bilirubin levels must be checked 4–6 hourly and the values plotted on a graph. If this suggests that the bilirubin will inevitably rise to > 350–360 µmol/l a further exchange transfusion is indicated, for which the baby should be transferred back to the NNU.

Before discharge, all rhesus babies must have their haemoglobin checked to ensure that they do not require a top-up transfusion. Their follow-up is described on p. 246.

OTHER BLOOD GROUP INCOMPATIBILITIES (RHESUS CcEe, KELl, DUFFY etc.)

The risk of HDN due to these antigens is also usually identified by antenatal screening of the mother. The incompatibility is confirmed in the neonate by testing cord blood which will show the appropriate blood group set-up and a positive direct Coombs' test (DCT). Most of these infants have a mild type of HDN, are often not anaemic or jaundiced when delivered, and can be managed on a postnatal ward. Some will never even become jaundiced since the haemolysis may be slow and the baby's liver may be able to cope with the bilirubin load. However, since they have a haemolytic problem, if jaundice does develop phototherapy should be started, and continued until the bilirubin is falling. They may also become anaemic, so careful follow-up is necessary (pp. 243–5).

UNANTICIPATED FIRST-DAY JAUNDICE

For babies whose first-day onset jaundice was *not* predicted on the basis of antenatal tests there are three likely haematological possibilities, though it is also important to exclude jaundice caused by infection on the first day as on any other (p. 298). The haematolgical causes are ABO HDN, spherocytosis and the non-spherocytic haemolytic anaemias (NSHA).

ABO incompatibility

Group A, B and most group O women have IgM isoagglutinins (anti-A, anti-B) which do not cross the placenta, but about 10 per cent of normal group O women and a smaller percentage of group A and B women have IgG anti-A haemolysin (and rarely anti-B) in their plasma which can cross the placenta and haemolyse the RBC of a group A infant (or rarely a group B one).

The antibody is present before pregnancy and so first babies may be affected. However, it is very unusual for the titres of these antibodies to rise as a result of feto-maternal bleeding at any stage of pregnancy and successive pregnancies are therefore rarely more severely affected than the first one.

In absolute numbers ABO HDN is 2–4 times more common than rhesus HDN. Fortunately, since the anti-A and anti-B haemolysins are comparatively weak antibodies, and much of the antibody which crosses the placenta is absorbed by A and B antigens in body tissues other than RBC, ABO HDN rarely causes severe problems.

ABO HDN usually presents in the first 24 hours of life, but it may also cause jaundice presenting on the third, fourth or fifth day of life. The haemoglobin is normal, and the DCT is either negative or weakly positive. The mother and baby are ABO incompatible. Proof of the diagnosis depends on identifying the haemolytic anti-A (or anti-B) haemolysins in maternal plasma or in the infant's plasma after eluting it from his RBC.

If this condition is recognised within the first 24–36 hours because of the rapid onset of jaundice, there is a distinct possibility that the bilirubin will rise to levels at which an exchange transfusion will be necessary. All such babies should, therefore, receive phototherapy once the diagnosis is established and this should be continued until the bilirubin is falling. The indications for exchange transfusion are given on p. 242.

Apart from jaundice, neonates with ABO HDN rarely have any other neonatal problems, but since they are more likely to become anaemic they should be followed up carefully (p. 246).

Spherocytosis

This often causes marked early onset neonatal jaundice and although an inherited disease, the family history has often been missed antenatally (p. 33). No specific treatment is required in the neonatal period other than management of the jaundice. The baby should be discharged on folic acid supplements, 1 mg o.d.

NSHA

These (e.g. glucose-6-phosphate dehydrogenase deficiency [G6PD], pyruvate kinase deficiency) should only be sought if HDN and spherocytosis have been excluded, unless the baby belongs to an ethnic group in which G6PD deficiency is likely (mainly blacks and those from countries around the Eastern Mediterranean). Their neonatal management, after taking blood for biochemical analysis, is that of the jaundice.

INFECTION

Sudden onset of jaundice at any stage in the neonatal period – on the first day, or even up to the third or fourth weeks – is an important marker of serious infection. Should jaundice develop in these circumstances, and particularly if there are any other features of infection (p. 294), the infant should be admitted to the neonatal unit for assessment.

PHYSIOLOGICAL JAUNDICE

For infants on a PNW this is by far and away the most common cause of neonatal jaundice. Compared with older children and adults, the neonate's liver is less efficient at binding bilirubin prior to conjugation, and is also less good at conjugating it. The more premature the baby, the greater is this problem.

In addition, the normal newborn is predisposed to jaundice for various reasons:

- His red cells have a shortened life span – 120 days in adults, 60–70 days at term, and about 40 days if premature.
- Polycythaemia, especially from placental transfusion (p. 75): delayed clamping of the cord increases the incidence of jaundice to over 30 per cent.
- Breakdown of bruises or RBC extravasated into tissues; this may be marked, for example following breech presentation, forceps delivery or with large cephalhaematomata.
- Dehydration and a hypocaloric intake in breast-fed babies before lactation is established (p. 139). This is a separate entity to the prolonged jaundice also seen in breast-fed infants which has a different aetiology (see below). Breast-fed infants, therefore, have two independent causes for an increased incidence of neonatal jaundice.
- Familial tendency.
- Conjugated bilirubin from the enterohepatic circulation (p. 232); the slower the intestinal transit time, the more bilirubin comes from this source.
- 'Shunt bilirubin' (20 per cent of the total), from

degradation of haem pigments synthesized in the marrow but never incorporated in to the circulating red cells.

Infants who become jaundiced for these reasons are those with so called 'physiological jaundice'.

Effects of drugs and obstetric practice

The incidence of neonatal jaundice is increased in babies delivered after induction of labour. Whether this is due to the drugs used for the induction, or whether it is some other effect of being induced such as instrumental delivery causing bruising, increased asphyxia, poor postnatal feeding and dehydration, varying the time when the cord is clamped, or simply an increase in the prematurity rate, remains unproven.

PROLONGED NEONATAL JAUNDICE

In the well term baby, by far and away the most common cause for this is breast-feeding. The aetiology is not yet established. Babies with breast milk jaundice thrive and gain weight at the approved rate of $30 \, g/24$ hours, and have no stigmata at all to suggest underlying liver disease. There is no hepatosplenomegaly, nor signs suggesting biliary obstruction, in particular the classical pale stools and a dark urine together with the presence of conjugated bilirubin in the plasma and urine. If other causes of unconjugated jaundice (Table 17.1) are suspected, they can usually easily be excluded on an out-patient basis. The bilirubin levels are usually in the $200-280 \, \mu mol/l$ range, and it is almost all unconjugated. After being static for 7–10 days these levels slowly fall, perhaps by no more than $5-10 \, \mu mol/day$, so that the baby can remain jaundiced for 6–8 weeks. The most important thing to remember about this condition is that it is benign and no treatment is required. The baby does not need to stop breast-feeding even for a day or two to establish the diagnosis by showing that the bilirubin rapidly falls on formula feeding.

TABLE 17.1 Causes of prolonged jaundice in the neonate

- Continuation of acute neonatal cause
  Haemolytic disease of the newborn*
  Infection*
- Breast-feeding
- Metabolic errors
  Galactosaemia*
  Hypothyroidism
  Tyrosinaemia*
  Fructosaemia
  Lucey-Driscoll syndrome (serum conjugation inhibitor)
  Crigler-Najjar syndrome
  Gilbert's disease
  Lipid storage diseases (e.g. Niemann Pick)
  Dubin-Johnson syndrome*
  Rotor syndrome*
- Hepatitis
  Congenital infection*
  Hepatitis
  Giant cell neonatal*
- Cystic fibrosis*
- Biliary atresia*
- α_1 antitrypsin deficiency*
- Biliary obstruction — bands, tumours, cysts*
- Prolonged i.v. feeding*

---

*There conditions may also cause obstructive jaundice.

Two serious (and treatable) causes of prolonged unconjugated jaundice are galactosaemia and hypothyroidism and these can be excluded easily, the former by testing the urine for sugar and the latter by the routine screening procedures (Chapter 9).

There is a long list of causes of prolonged neonatal jaundice (Table 17.1) most of which are extremely rare or untreatable. However, appropriate tests should always be carried out. If biliary atresia is suspected on the basis of a conjugated hyperbilirubinaemia, hepatomegaly, pale stools and dark urine, assessment is urgent since successful surgery is only likely if it is carried out before the age of 6–7 weeks. However, this diagnosis is rarely suspected, never mind established, until after the baby has gone home from the maternity hospital.

INVESTIGATION

Mild jaundice, thought to be physiological, does not need to be investigated, and furthermore, with a little practice a physician can judge clinically those milder degrees of jaundice in which it is not even necessary to measure the plasma bilirubin. These skills, however, should not be relied upon on coloured babies, in particular black ones, in whom it is exceptionally difficult to assess jaundice clinically. In such infants, therefore, if any degree of jaundice is suspected clinically, the exact levels should be established biochemically.

Once the plasma bilirubin rises above $200 \, \mu mol/l$ the baby should have his plasma bilirubin checked at least daily until the level is falling, or it is clear that it is stable and not going to rise to $> 300–350 \, \mu mol/l$.

However, if the plasma bilirubin in the baby with 'physiological jaundice' rises above $270 \, \mu mol/l$ (16 mg%), bearing in mind the injunction on p. 234 that jaundice should alert the paediatrician to seek its cause, the investigations in Table 17.2 should be carried out, and appropriate treatment given if the investigations are positive.

TABLE 17.2   Investigation of asymptomatic jaundiced neonates

Investigation	Comment
Urinalysis	Occult UTI (p. 223)
WBC and differential	Good marker of occult infection
Blood group, Coombs' test	Milder end of blood group incompatibility illness
G6PD assay	Appropriate ethnic group (black, Mediterranean)

TREATMENT OF NEONATAL JAUNDICE

Apart from babies with rhesus (D) incompatibility, most neonates described in this chapter will not need exchange transfusion unless the bilirubin exceeds 350–375 µmol/l in babies 34–37 weeks gestation and 425–430 µmol/l in those >37 weeks (see Fig. 17.2).

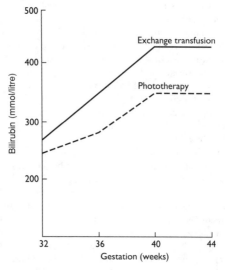

FIGURE 17.2 Action lines for treating neonatal jaundice in well babies.

ADEQUATE HYDRATION

In the jaundice seen in breast-fed infants in the first 3–4 days (p. 138) an element of dehydration and under-feeding may occur particularly if the weight loss exceeds 8–10 per cent. In these babies increase the frequency of breast-feeds to 2–3 hourly, consider giving the mother Maxolon (p. 156), but only give complementary feeds of 10 per cent dextrose (p. 163) if the bilirubin rises to more than $340\,\mu mol/l$, test weighing shows that the mother is producing very little milk, and an exchange transfusion is looming. Consider using formula, since there is some evidence to suggest that glucose feeds may make the baby more yellow.

DRUGS

The enzymes of bilirubin glucuronidation can be induced by various drugs, in particular phenobarbitone. However, it takes 48 hours for the drug to have any effect, and phenobarbitone makes the infant sleepy and feed poorly. This therapy has no place in current neonatal practice except in the management of Crigler-Najjar syndrome.

Although laxatives also lower neonatal serum bilirubin, their use is not justified even though it is often noted that the jaundice in pre-term infants only starts to clear once they have had their bowels open.

PHOTOTHERAPY

There are three methods by which phototherapy reduces the amount of unconjugated bilirubin in the plasma (Roberton, 1986):

- Photoisomerization of the bilirubin to produce a non-toxic but yellow isomer.
- Intramolecular cyclisation between adjacent pyrrole rings: this also produces a non-toxic but yellow isomer called lumirubin.
- Photo-oxidation to colourless pyrollic and dipyrollic compounds.

As soon as phototherapy is started, it is important to recognise that even though the total bilirubin as measured by the bilirubinometer stays constant, some of it (15–20 per cent) is present as these yellow photo-isomers which are not neurotoxic.

Indications

In controlled trials in rhesus (D) haemolytic disease phototherapy halves the number of second or subsequent exchange transfusion carried out and it should always be used in such infants. The other indications for phototherapy on a postnatal ward are:

- Jaundiced babies with ABO or other blood group incompat-ibilities, or with RBC abnormalities, e.g. spherocytosis, until it is clear that exchangetransfusion will not be indicated and the bilirubin is falling.
- Bilirubin levels 250–360 μmol/l (15–20 mg%) in healthy infants, using the lower level in neonates nearer 32 weeks and the upper level in babies of 40 weeks (Fig. 17.1).

Do not give phototherapy for conjugated jaundice, since the babies are likely to turn a deep brown colour probably due to photodegradation of porphyrins in the plasma of infants with conjugated hyperbilirubinaemia.

No serious long-term sequelae of phototherapy have been reported; however phototherapy:

- Decreases gut transit time, i.e. loose stools develop, probably due to the irritant effect on the bowel of the photoisomers of bilirubin.
- Increases fluid loss through the skin and gut.
- Exposes the neonate to the risks of hypo- and hyperthermia.
- Causes erythematous rashes.

However, probably the most serious adverse effect of phototherapy is the anxiety it provokes in the mothers who have their baby removed, blindfolded and laid naked under a bright light. The technique should, therefore, only be used if really indicated.

Management of phototherapy

- Do it in the postnatal ward beside the mother if the baby is otherwise well and weighs more than 1.80 kg.

- Keep the baby as free from clothing as possible. Many infants are covered with nappies, hats, bootees, blindfolds and bits of sticky tape holding on various monitors, with the result that little light reaches the skin.

- Take great care with the thermal environment: naked babies in a cool room may become hypothermic.

- Watch the fluid balance: phototherapy may double the fluid loss through a small baby's skin and gut, appropriate increases in fluid intake may be necessary.

- Blindfold him, but be careful that this does not cause conjunctivitis due to irritation from the bandaging.

- Check the irradiance of the lights every 100–200 hours of use to ensure that they are still effective. Their radiance should be greater than $4\,\mu W/cm^2/nm$; if it is not, the bulbs should be replaced.

- **Do not give it unnecessarily.**

Stopping phototherapy

In all jaundiced neonates, even those with a haemolytic jaundice, the phototherapy can be stopped as soon as the bilirubin plateaus or begins to fall. If it starts to climb again, restart phototherapy, though this is rarely necessary. Once the bilirubin is falling, persisting clinically apparent jaundice is not a reason *per se* for keeping a baby in hospital.

FOLLOW-UP

With any baby treated on a postnatal ward for neonatal jaundice, the assumption should be that sequelae are going to be the exception rather than the rule. There are, therefore, two groups of babies who need follow-up:

- Those in whom the phototherapy was given for a haemolytic jaundice, e.g. rhesus HDN, ABO HDN, G6PD deficiency. Neonates with rhesus(D) incompatibility should take iron and folic acid at home for 2–3 months, and be carefully followed up at weekly or two weekly intervals after discharge to ensure that they do not become anaemic (haemoglobin < 7–8 g%, in which case a top-up transfusion is needed). Follow-up should continue in these neonates until the haemoglobin is rising spontaneously or maintained > 9 g%. Infants with other blood group incompatibilities rarely need supplements, but should be checked 2–4 weeks after discharge to make sure that an anaemia has not developed.

In those with an underlying red cell defect such as spherocytosis or G6PD deficiency long-term follow-up is indicated.

- Babies, virtually always breast-fed, who are still moderately jaundiced at discharge, and in whom reliance cannot be placed on the mother or the primary care services to take appropriate action in the rare event of the jaundice persisting. Particular care should be taken to identify those with features of obstructive jaundice (pale stools, dark urine, hepatosplenomegaly) and/or with failure to thrive which might indicate hepatitis or biliary atresia. These babies should be referred urgently to hospital for further investigation.

REFERENCES

McClure, G. (1992). Haemolytic disease of the newborn. In: *Textbook of Neonatology*, 2nd Ed. Ed. N.R.C. Roberton. Churchill Livingstone, Edinburgh, London, 725–732.

Roberton, N.R.C. (1986). Neonatal jaundice. In: *Recent Advances in Paediatrics*. No. 8. Ed. Meadow, R. Churchill Livingstone, Edinburgh, London, 157–184.

Roberton, N.R.C. (1993). *A Manual of Neonatal Intensive Care*, 3rd Ed. Edward Arnold, London.

18

COMMON PROBLEMS IN THE WELL NEONATE

—

CAPUT SUCCEDANEUM/MOULDING

Babies who have been in labour for a long time may have marked elongation of their heads due to moulding of the skull bones plus subcutaneous oedema, with the apex of the elongation over the area of the posterior fontanelle (the vertex). It may be markedly bruised as well. No matter how large, this is a benign condition which will recede over the first 2–3 days. The name of the condition is usually abbreviated to *caput*. The absence of caput in babies presenting by the breech gives them a different head shape from the vast majority of vertex presenting babies. This may cause anxiety in inexperienced nurses or physicians. A measurement of the head circumference (OFC, p. 96) taken in the presence of a caput is clearly of little value as a base line measurement of the head size.

The moulding and bruising which occurs with a face or brow presentation, even if the mother was eventually delivered by caesarean section, may be very striking and distort the infant's facial appearance. However, no action is required, and the swelling settles within 2–3 days.

VENTOUSE, CHIGNON

The scalp tissues underneath the site of application of a Ventouse cup are sucked into the cup with the application of the vacuum. This results in a raised purplish oedematous lump of scalp known as a chignon. Like the caput, this alarming protuberance is benign and can be allowed to settle spontaneously, and will do so over the first 3–4 days.

CEPHALHAEMATOMA

This is a subperiosteal accumulation of blood usually lying over one or both parietal bones, but occasionally over the frontal or occipital bones. Because it is limited by the periosteum, the swelling of a cephalhaematoma never crosses a suture line. Older data suggests that cephalhaematomata were commonly associated with a small underlying linear skull fracture. This is not a lesion that should be sought, since it never causes medical problems, but it clearly may arouse considerable parental anxiety if not legal problems.

A large cephalhaematoma can contain 10–15 ml of blood, and the 1.5–2.0 g of haemoglobin which this contains has to be broken down, yielding 900–1200 μmol of bilirubin which therefore increases the likelihood of the neonate developing jaundice (p. 238). No treatment is required for cephalhaematomata. They must never be aspirated since this merely introduces infection. Occasionally, if there is an underlying haemorrhagic disorder the cephalhaematoma may continue to increase in size after delivery. If this happens, correction of the coagulation disturbance is the correct treatment. As cephalhaematomata resorb, a ridge of bone may form round their periphery giving the illusion of a depressed central area. Always reassure the mother that this lesion is harmless, and that the lump will resolve completely, and that her baby will have a beautifully smooth skull.

SUBGALEAL HAEMORRHAGE

A rare lesion, more common in but not restricted to black babies, and in particular those not given prophylactic vitamin K, is a large subgaleal haemorrhage (the blood lying between the cranial aponeurosis and periosteum). This develops in the first 2–3 days, and can obviously cover the whole of the scalp which feels boggy, and often has an odd, loose feel to it. The haemorrhage may be so large that the condition occasionally presents with the baby in haemorrhagic shock. No specific treatment is indicated except for treating the anaemia which may require transfusion, and for the jaundice which usually results from the breakdown of the large amount of blood in the haemorrhage. The lesion spontaneously resolves over the first 2–3 weeks of life.

CUTS, BRUISES AND ABRASIONS

The baby may be cut during a caesarean section, and bruising of varying degrees is common whenever the delivery was difficult. Any form of manual manipulation will cause bruising, more so in pre-term babies. Striking bruising of the presenting part – legs, buttocks and genitalia – is seen with a breech delivery, and after the use of forceps there may be marked facial bruising outlining the site of application of the forceps blades over the baby's face and head. The application of fetal scalp clips, or the taking of fetal scalp samples, may cause surprisingly large cuts and holes in the baby's scalp.

These lesions should all be treated on their merit. Cuts can usually be closed with Steristrip, although, occasionally, suturing is necessary. Abrasions should be kept dry and clean, and are usually best managed by exposure. Bruising requires no active treatment, even when it is spectacular and involves the external genitalia of either sex following breech delivery, but it does considerably increase the likelihood of the baby developing moderate to severe jaundice (p. 238).

TRAUMATIC CYANOSIS

Babies who have been difficult vaginal deliveries, often have marked facial and/or scalp congestion with petechiae. The condition is called traumatic cyanosis, and its major importance is that it should not be confused with central cyanosis, thereby raising the possibility of lung or heart disease. Traumatic cyanosis requires no treatment and fades within 48–72 hours.

PUFFY EYELIDS

Many neonates have extremely puffy upper and lower lids during the first 2–3 days – probably a localisation of the oedema seen with a caput or from the pressure which causes traumatic cyanosis. The mother is often disturbed because the baby never opens his eyes. No action is required, and the mother can be reassured that the swelling will recede and the baby open his eyes by the third or fourth day.

SUBCONJUNCTIVAL HAEMORRHAGE

The same forces as those which cause cephal-haematomata, traumatic cyanosis and puffy eyelids may also result in subconjunctival haemorrhage in the newborn baby. The haemorrhages are often quite striking on both sides of the iris, but are always benign. The mother can be reassured.

FRACTURES

Clavicle

This is the most common neonatal fracture, and occurs either during delivery of the shoulders in a breech extraction, or more commonly when there is difficulty delivering the anterior shoulder (shoulder dystocia) of a large baby presenting by the vertex. A crack may be heard as the bone snaps; alternatively, the injury may present either in the first 48 hours when a lump (callus) is noted over the collar bone, or during the evaluation of a neonate with the frequently associated Erb's palsy (v.i.). In general no treatment is required for the fracture. If the baby appears to be in pain, which is surprisingly rare, he can be placed in a figure of eight bandage, though this is rarely necessary for more than 7–10 days. The mother can be reassured that the fracture will heal with no subsequent deformity.

Humerus

This can be fractured when delivering the intravaginal arm of a breech. A crack may be heard, and the radial nerve may be damaged as it traverses the spiral groove of the humerus. If not recognised at delivery, the lesion is often detected within the first two days because of reduced and painful movements of the arm, and if the radial nerve was damaged, by a paucity of hand movements. The X-ray may show marked displacement and angulation. Treatment, however, is simple splinting to reduce pain, by putting the baby in a long-sleeved nightshirt and pinning the sleeve to the chest, or by loosely bandaging his arm against his thorax. This splinting should be maintained usually for 2–3 weeks, and complete neurological and orthopaedic recovery is the rule without any shortening or angulation of the bone.

Forearm bones, femur

These can be broken, again, during the manoeuvres involved in a vaginal breech delivery. If an audible intrapartum crack does not result in the recognition of the injury, the infant usually presents with reduced and painful movements of the affected limb. Femoral fractures may be more markedly displaced and angulated, but no treatment is necessary other than splinting for 3–4 weeks in a plaster of Paris cast, and complete recovery is the rule. Forearm fractures recover with no therapy other than supporting bandage to reduce pain.

FACIAL NERVE PALSY (BELL'S PALSY, VII NERVE PALSY)

This is usually the result of compression of the facial nerve against the mandibular ramus during a forceps delivery. It is, therefore, a lower motor neurone lesion reducing the movements round the eye and mouth. In the vast majority of cases, it is transient, lasting < 1–2 hours in some cases, and most recover within 24–36 hours.

If a baby presents with a VII nerve palsy without the forceps being applied, this suggests either that the nerve was compressed between the mandible and some part of the maternal pelvis for some period pre- or intrapartum, or that there is a central problem, often with dysgenesis of the VII nerve nucleus. In the latter group the lesion is often associated with other cranial nerves palsies (III,IV,V,VI) which will be apparent on examination. The prognosis for the former is poor, and is inversely proportional to the duration of facial nerve compression pre-delivery; a permanent defect is likely in the latter. Nevertheless, jaw and mouth movements and feeding are rarely compromised. Plastic surgery to prevent injuries to the cornea of the non-closing eye may be necessary.

BRACHIAL PLEXUS PALSY

This is usually an Erb's palsy in which the upper roots of the brachial plexus are involved (C5,6,7) causing weakness of the shoulder muscles, the biceps, brachioradialis and the supinators of the forearm. The affected arm moves poorly and lies in the typical 'waiter's tip' position (Fig. 18.1), which is readily recognised from clinical observation, and demon-

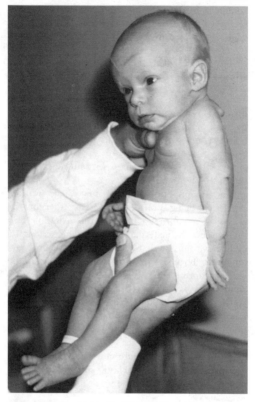

FIGURE 18.1 Baby with left side Erb's palsy. The arm is hanging limply in the 'waiter's tip' position (from Hensinger and Jones, 1992, with permission).

strated more dramatically by the Moro response (p. 100). In some cases the phrenic nerve may also be involved, and in severe injuries the lower roots of the brachial plexus will be damaged (C8, T1), paralysing the small muscles of the forearm and hand as well (Klumpke's paralysis).

The injury is caused by traction on the nerve roots when the head and shoulder are pulled apart. This is the same traction force which causes a fractured clavicle with which it frequently co-exists (v.s.). In most cases, the roots are merely stretched or have a haematoma round them which causes nerve compression. Complete disruption of the roots is rare. No treatment is indicated initially, since in most cases the swelling caused by the trauma or haemorrhage resolves, and neurological function rapidly returns. The longer the physical signs of Erb's palsy persist, the greater the likelihood that there has been total disruption of the nerve roots, and the poorer the long-term prognosis; babies with marked limitation of movement by 7–10 days are unlikely to make a full recovery. In such babies, gentle physiotherapy should be instituted at this stage to prevent contractures, particularly around the shoulder joint, adding to the restricted mobility of the nerve palsy. Surgical correction of the torn plexus has been described, and should be considered if the paralysis remains dense after one month.

NEUROLOGICAL PROBLEMS

DISORDERS OF TONE

Problems in assessing tone are alluded to on p. 97. Most neonates with marked abnormality in tone are ill, on the NNICU, and usually have serious underlying neurological problems.

In babies on a PNW, hypotonia may be the presenting feature of severe acute neonatal illness, in particular all forms of sepsis, and the severe inborn errors of metabolism characterised by organic acidaemia or hyperammonaemia (p. 292). If a floppy infant seems ill as well as floppy, he should be transferred at once to the NNICU, but if abnormalities of tone are detected in an otherwise apparently well neonate the possibilities outlined below should be considered. In general these all cause hypotonia, though occasionally hypertonia may be seen in dysmorphic syndromes.

• **Maternal pregnancy history:**	
Severe maternal illness, maternal drug therapy or abuse (pp. 16–52)	Can cause permanent fetal CNS damage
• **Intrapartum history**:	
Use of analgesics, sedatives, anticonvulsants	Drug depression of the neonate or mild hypoxic ischaemic encephalopathy;
Low Apgar score	These are the most common cause of neonatal hypotonia
• **Maternal examination**:	
Myotonia, myopathic facies, i.e. dystrophia myotonica; myasthenia	Neonatal dystrophia myotonica; neonatal myasthenia
• **Clinical examination of the neonate**:	
Evidence of weakness as well as hypotonia (not moving against gravity, mouth hanging open)	Suggests primary neurological or muscle disorder
Tongue fasciculation	A marker of Werdnig-Hoffman disease
Abnormal dysmorphic features	Check against the atlases (p. 309)

In most cases, no abnormality other than the hypotonia (hypertonia) will be found, and the abnormality of tone is usually attributed to intrapartum drug therapy or the sequelae of mild birth asphyxia. All that is required in such a baby is the occasional tube feed to tide him over the next 24–48 hours by which time his problem resolves.

If no diagnosis has been made, but marked hypotonia persists, consider neonatal myasthenia by doing a Tensilon test,* and exclude intracranial problems by cranial ultrasound. If necessary, proceed to muscle biopsy and CT scan, but these should only be carried out in a centre with appropriate expertise.

ENLARGED FONTANELLE, WIDE SUTURES

So long as the baby's OFC is appropriate for his birthweight, and there are no other clinical abnormalities, no action is necessary (p. 96); if in doubt, cranial ultrasound is readily available, easily performed and totally safe, and will virtually always be normal in a baby with a normal OFC no matter how large the fontanelle and sutures. If the separation is very marked but the baby is otherwise neurologically normal consider primary bone disorders, e.g. osteogenesis imperfecta.

ABNORMAL CRY

Feeble cries usually go with floppy, feeble babies and should be evaluated accordingly. The feeble mewing cry of the Cri-du-Chat syndrome (deletion of short arm of chromosome 5 [5p-]) will occur in 1:100 000 neonates, and the diagnosis can be confirmed by chromosome analysis.

The high pitched cry of neonatal meningitis is a late sign of the disease implying that earlier indications of severe sepsis were missed (p. 297). It should never be heard in a well-run unit.

Babies who are described as 'cerebral' or 'jittery' or 'irritable' (see below) often have a particularly ear-piercing howl.

IRRITABLE, CEREBRAL BABIES

A well recognised neonate is the one, often large, commonly produced by a difficult forceps delivery or by the breech, who is difficult to feed, cries piercingly, is difficult to soothe by cuddling, and sleeps fitfully.

---

*Give 1mg of edrophonium chloride i.m.; the muscle tone in neonates with myasthenia will dramatically improve.

This is one of the milder aftermaths of intrapartum cerebral hypoxia and can be considered to be grade I hypoxic ischaemic encephalopathy. So long as the baby is otherwise neurologically normal, and feeds to some extent, he should be swaddled and kept peaceful. Activities other than feeding which result in the baby being prodded, stimulated or woken should be reduced to the absolute minimum. Pharmacological sedation in such babies is contraindicated as it makes them floppy and more difficult to feed, and in reasonable (as opposed to anaesthetic) doses does no more than can be achieved by peace, quiet and swaddling. These babies will settle down in the first 2–3 days, and have no long-term sequelae.

JITTERY BABIES

Jitteriness is a high-frequency (about 10/second) low-amplitude 'tremulous' movement caused by rapid rhythmic contraction of opposing muscle groups (as opposed to the rapid contraction of flexor muscles followed by their slow relaxation which is the movement seen in a clonic fit). It is characteristically seen in SFD infants (though it is probably no more frequent in those with a low glucose than with a normal blood glucose), with hypocalcaemia and in the irritable cerebral babies alluded to above. In general no treatment is required other than tranquillity and swaddling. The management of smallness-for-dates is outlined in Chapter 11.

In larger jittery babies a single Dextrostix can be done to allay medical neurosis by confirming the absence of hypoglycaemia. If jitteriness is marked and persistent, it may be worth measuring the calcium and giving calcium supplements (p. 280) in the rare baby in whom hypocalcaemia is documented.

EYES

Subconjunctival haemorrhages
(p. 251)

Squint

Most babies cross their eyes and roll them around in a most alarming fashion. So long as these are the usually transient abnormalities of ocular movement, no investigation is required. A fixed squint needs further evaluation by careful clinical examination, and usually by a cranial ultrasound. A VI nerve palsy can occur following a difficult delivery, and usually resolves rapidly. Other lesions are rare, and usually the result of severe birth asphyxia or an underlying neurological malformation.

RESPIRATORY SYSTEM

A baby with any respiratory symptom – coughing, choking, apnoea, cyanosis or tachy- or dyspnoea – usually requires admission to the neonatal unit.

STRIDOR

Some babies who required intubation for resuscitation after delivery, or in whom blind oro-pharyngeal suction was too vigorous, develop transient respiratory stridor, usually only when crying, in the first 2–3 days. It is presumably due to mild traumatic pharyngeal and laryngeal oedema. If the stridor is persistent, or causes any respiratory distress, the neonate's upper airway should be examined by direct laryngoscopy.

NASAL DEFORMITY

Many babies, even without incorrectly applied forceps, can be born with quite marked distortion of the nasal septum, primarily due to the nose being pressed against part of the maternal pelvis. No action is required, and the noses show a remarkable capacity for spontaneous straightening.

CARDIAC PROBLEMS

One of the most frustrating features of neonatal cardiology is that most babies with murmurs or abnormal findings on the first 1–2 days do *not* have cardiac disease. Conversely, and more worrying, most babies with serious or fatal congenital heart disease will have no abnormalities on routine first-day examination (pp. 90–3).

ABNORMALITIES OF PULSE

An irregular pulse, and a pulse rate consistently < 90/min or > 180/min always merit an ECG. If abnormalities other than sinus bradycardia or tachycardia are found (the exception rather than the rule), further assessment including an echocardiogram may be necessary.

Although some entirely normal babies have a sinus bradycardia of 80–90/min and probably do not need further assessment, a persisting sinus tachycardia is abnormal and requires assessment.

Common causes include:
- systemic illness, especially infection;
- heart failure;
- pyrexia, over-heating or infection;
- drugs, e.g. theophylline;
- thyrotoxicosis.

Supaventricular tachycardias, usually with a pulse rate > 200, need pharmacological control.

MURMURS

Hearing a murmur is one of the most common findings on the routine neonatal clinical examination (p. 91) and may be present in 60–80 per cent of neonates examined in the first 24 hours of life. However, the incidence of congenital heart disease is a hundredth of this, i.e. about 6–8:1000 live births. It is essential, therefore, not to over-react to the presence of a murmur in a way that will result in over-investigation of the baby and provoke unnecessary parental anxiety.

If a murmur is found on examination of a neonate, a watching brief is indicated if:

- The baby is < 48–72 hours old, he is pink and otherwise completely asymptomatic, with no dyspnoea, no signs of heart failure, normal pulses and feeding well.
- At any age if the murmur is short, and mid-systolic ≤ 2/6, and the rest of the examination is normal.

In such cases, in the first 24–48 hours it is reasonable not to frighten the parents by telling them about the murmur, but to return and check the baby at 48–72 hours of age. Investigation which should include echocardiography in most cases is, however, indicated if:

- The above criteria do not apply.
- The murmur 'sounds significant', is pansystolic or spills into diastole, there is a separate diastolic murmur, there is a thrill, or other signs of heart disease are present including, of course, cyanosis and heart failure.

The signs of heart failure are:

- increased respiratory rate, increased heart rate, triple rhythm (S3 present);
- cardiomegaly – difficult to assess clinically, but seen on CXR;
- pulmonary crepitations (left ventricular failure);
- hepatosplenomegaly;
- sweating, clammy baby;
- raised JVP (very difficult to see in the neonate);
- weight gain > 15 mg/kg/24 hours (a very useful indicator);
- peripheral oedema (a late sign);

- remember that heart failure may be caused by an extracardiac shunt (p. 92). The management of the neonate with serious heart disease is outlined on pp. 290–1.

Follow-up

If a baby has a soft mid-systolic noise on discharge from the PNW, the parents must obviously be informed. There are two management options. One is to reassure them (correctly) that the murmur will probably disappear, do no investigations, arrange follow-up in 2–4 weeks and investigate sometime later only the small proportion with persisting signs. The other is to do a CXR and echocardiogram on them all, and establish the diagnosis which in many cases will be either a spontaneously recovering lesion such as a small VSD or 'normal heart'. My own preference is for the former.

MOUTH

TONGUE

Tongue abnormalities are rare in the neonate. An oddly shaped tongue, or a tongue and gums with lumps and bumps, may be part of a syndrome complex. Refer to the catalogues (p. 309).

Tongue tie

The length and thickness of the frenulum from the tongue to the floor of the mouth varies considerably. Those with short thick frenulae are said to have 'tongue tie'. Most paediatricians, including this one, believe that this is a normal finding and in particular that it never causes feeding or speech problems.

Some surgeons think differently; they should be kept away from the baby.

TEETH

These may be present, and are usually incisors; there are rarely more than two and they are always loose. They should be removed. The primary dentition will still be normal, and will appear at the normal time.

RANULAE

These are mucous inclusion cysts in the sublingual salivary glands on the floor of the infant's mouth. They are usually small, can be ignored and will spontaneously regress. Larger ones need surgical removal.

PALATE

Small mid-line posterior clefts are often missed until the routine neonatal clinical examination (p. 94). The management of harelip and cleft palate is described on pp. 312–3. White inclusion cysts 1–3 mm in diameter (Epstein's Pearls – the intra-oral equivalent of milia (p. 281)) are often noted on the hard palate. They are inconsequential and disappear. An abnormally shaped palate, high arched or irregular, and lumps and bumps on the gums, may be part of a syndrome (see the catalogues, p. 309), but if it is an isolated finding, no further action is required.

EPULIS

This is the name given to a benign tumour comprising vascular connective tissue arising from the gums or mouth. It may protrude from the mouth, and should always be removed.

GASTROINTESTINAL TRACT

HAEMATEMESIS

The most common cause of haematemesis in the first 48 hours is maternal blood swallowed by the baby during delivery; after 48 hours, it is maternal blood from a cracked nipple swallowed by a breast-fed baby. The maternal origin can be confirmed by Apt's test.* Once the maternal origin of the blood has been established, no further action, from the baby's point of view at least, is necessary.

In the previously healthy neonate, there are only two likely causes of haematemesis of neonatal blood: trauma or haemorrhagic disease. The infant's airway may have been injured by suction or intubation during resuscitation, or his GI tract may occasionally have been damaged by either a misplaced endotracheal tube during resuscitation, or by passing a nasogastric tube to feed him.

Haemorrhagaic disease is virtually limited to babies who have not been given vitamin K prophylaxis and may be the presentation of this condition. Using Apt's test the blood will be found to be neonatal. Since the baby may have had a large haemorrhage, give him 1 mg of vitamin K intramuscularly stat, after sending a sample of his blood to check the level of the clotting factors. He should then be transferred at once to the neonatal unit.

It is exceptionally rare for haematemesis to occur for reasons other than these in a previously well term baby. However, if more than a few millilitres of neonatal blood is vomited, and there is no history of trauma (e.g. nasogastric tubes), it is safer to admit the baby to the NNICU, check his coagulation status and watch carefully for signs of further haemorrhage (p. 301).

ABNORMAL STOOL COLOUR

Mothers read great things in to the colour of their babies' motions; paediatricians should not. Blood and

---

*Apt's test: add 1ml of 1% NaOH to 1ml of a dilute solution of the bloody effluent in water: fetal haemoglobin stays pink, whereas adult haemoglobin denatures and goes brown.

melaena are clearly important (see below); very pale stools in a jaundiced baby may imply biliary obstruction, and that is also serious. Other than these features stool colour is of doubtful importance. Green stools in particular cause alarm. The greenness may be oral iron therapy, and is often attributed to 'hunger stools'. However, undernutrition is better assessed by weighing the baby and seeing how he feeds.

MELAENA

In most neonates with melaena the aetiology is the same as for haematemesis – swallowed maternal blood. Apt's test is less reliable on melaena than on haematemesis, and if there is any doubt about the diagnosis, haemorrhagic disease should be assumed, blood sent for coagulation studies, vitamin K given and the infant admitted to the NNICU for observation. Melaena may also be due to some gastrointestinal tract malformation of the sort that more often causes fresh bleeding PR (v.i.), and these should be sought if melaena is persistent, and none of the above causes are found.

BLEEDING PR

Commonly, the appearance of fresh blood PR is due either to local trauma or a fissure-in-ano. The infant's rectum can be traumatised by thermometers, or by the large fingers of a clinician who does a rectal examination. Fissure-in-ano is a small tear in the anal margin probably caused by passing hard stools. It can occur anywhere on the margin, but is usually at 6 or 12 o'clock, and it is easily diagnosed by inspection and gently retracting the buttocks. No treatment is usually required in the neonate other than increasing the fluid intake so that the stools become softer; healing then occurs within 2–3 days.

Bleeding PR, usually fresh blood, but it can be

melaena, can be the first sign of serious neonatal bowel disease such as intussusception, colitis or necrotising enterocolitis as well as malformations such as polyps or a Meckel's diverticulum. If there is no history of trauma, clotting studies are normal and the anal margin is normal (see above), these conditions must be sought by careful examination in the first place, and followed by a plain X-ray and an abdominal ultrasound scan. Most such babies will need admission to the NNICU for further investigation.

VOMITING

The first thing the physician must always do when given the history of neonatal vomiting is to ascertain its severity. It is very common and entirely normal for babies to bring up a small amount of, usually curdled, milk. This can happen at any time after a feed, may be frequent and often coincides with the baby being 'winded' (pp. 160–1). Although the amount produced rarely covers more than a few square inches of the sheet or the baby's clothing, it is smelly and messy, and commonly arouses more maternal anxiety than any other symptom arising in the neonatal period. Nevertheless, if the baby appears normal on clinical examination, if his weight is normal and the vomit contains no bile or blood the mother can be reassured that many babies do just vomit.

Immediately after birth, vomiting is often attributed to having swallowed maternal blood or meconium, or to the infant being 'mucousy'. In these situations the vomiting is purported to respond to a stomach wash-out using 10–20 ml aliquots of 2.5 per cent $NaHCO_3$. The value of this procedure is, in my view, doubtful, but it certainly provides harmless psychotherapy for the nurses and the mother.

Non-bilious vomiting

If non-bilious vomiting is persistent in the first 24–48

hours, a high intestinal obstruction, usually duodenal atresia, must be excluded by the appropriate plain erect abdominal X-ray (see Chapter 19).

Persistent vomiting after the first 3–4 days is unusual in the absence of features of intestinal obstruction (p. 300). If the infant is ill, it usually indicates infection (p. 297), or gastroenteritis (p. 225–6) and the infant should be appropriately managed. Later in the neonatal period the common causes of vomiting in infancy should be considered; these include:

- upper respiratory tract infection;
- otitis media;
- urinary tract infection;
- pyloric stenosis;
- hiatus hernia, regurgitation.

Most of these conditions are rare in the neonatal period, though many mothers of babies who present later in infancy with 'posseting' and regurgitation due to the last diagnosis, date the onset of symptoms to the neonatal period. In persistent vomiting in the neonatal period, barium studies may be indicated as a last resort, to rule out rare causes of sub-acute intestinal obstruction.

Bilious vomiting

In the presence of bilious vomiting, the diagnosis is intestinal obstruction until proved otherwise, and the neonate should be admitted to the neonatal unit for evaluation. However, a few entirely normal babies can have a spell of bilious vomiting in the neonatal period (Lilien *et al.*, 1986).

It must be emphasised that in the absence of signs of infection, obstruction or bloody vomiting, 99.9 per cent of 'sicky' babies settle down with nothing more than a stomach wash-out and patience. There is absolutely no need to change a baby's formula, or worse still abandon breast-feeding, just because he vomits.

FAILURE TO PASS MECONIUM

Genuine failure to pass meconium (i.e. the fact that meconium was passed intrapartum has not been forgotten) by 48 hours of age in an otherwise entirely normal term baby on a PNW is always abnormal. It should be regarded as an absolute indication to exclude Hirschsprung's disease by rectal biopsy unless some other condition such as meconium plug or meconium ileus can be established by clinical or radiological examinations. Failure to pass meconium before 48 hours can be managed by observing the baby and waiting for things to happen.

ABDOMINAL DISTENSION

The pathological causes of abdominal distension are outlined on p. 299, and the cause is usually easily established by getting a history suggesting intestinal obstruction, or by finding that one of the intra-abdominal viscera is enlarged. If, as is usually the case, these features are absent, the baby should be carefully observed on the PNW, with the expectation that he will turn out to be entirely normal.

DIASTASIS RECTI

In many normal neonates the two sheaths of the rectus abdominis do not meet at the linea alba so that when the infant strains there is a fusiform bulge through the mid-line of the abdominal wall. This disappears during the first year as the rectus sheath closes up. The mother can be reassured.

INGUINAL HERNIA

These are rare in the full term neonate. If present, they usually need to be operated on. In girls they should raise the suspicion that the mass in the sac is a testicle, and you are dealing with a case of testicular feminisation syndrome.

UMBILICAL PROBLEMS

Care of the umbilical cord is described on pp. 75–6 and infection on p. 222. A very small amount of bleeding as the cord separates is common, but anything more than a few spots requires careful observation; haemostasis (pressure for 5–10 minutes is usually adequate) and vitamin K i.m. if this had not been given.

Rarely, a very small omphalocoele may be detected later in the neonatal period, or urine may be found dribbling from a patent urachus. Surgical referral is indicated.

Umbilical hernia

These occur more commonly in black than white babies. A small defect in the linea alba usually < 1 cm diameter, covered with peritoneum and skin only, can be felt under the umbilical stump. Although these herniae may become very large, they hardly ever incarcerate, never mind strangulate. In the rare case in whom the defect does not spontaneously close by 1–2 years of age, surgery may be indicated, but should not be carried out before then.

Umbilical granuloma

Occasionally, after the cord has separated, a granuloma develops over the area of necrotic Wharton's jelly at the centre of the umbilicus; it may be friable and bleed. After ensuring that it is not an omphalocoele or connected to a urachal remnant, the lesion should be rubbed with a silver nitrate stick, taking care not to burn surrounding skin, and it will rapidly disappear.

GENITOURINARY PROBLEMS

HAEMATURIA

This usually means that something pink was found in the nappy – and it is commonly salmon pink urate crystals; in girls it may be vaginal blood (v.i.). Genuine haematuria in the neonate is rare, and if there is no local trauma, always pathological, demanding investigation by clinical examination, urine analysis, coagulation screening (since disseminated intravascular coagulation is probably the most common cause) and by renal and bladder ultrasound to exclude malformations.

Most babies with haematuria are either ill or have a malformation which will need surgery, and they should, therefore, be admitted to the NNU.

HYDROCOELE

The fluctuant, transilluminating swelling of a hydrocoele is common and harmless, irrespective of its size. The mother should be reassured.

TORSION

A hard tender mass in the neonate's scrotum is almost always a testicular torsion and requires urgent assessment, and usually an operation. However, even if this is arranged immediately, it is rarely possible to preserve the testis as a functional organ. To prevent a similar fate befalling the contralateral testis it should always be tethered in the scrotum at operation.

UNDESCENDED TESTES

Three per cent of term male babies have one or both testes missing on routine neonatal clinical examination. Nothing needs to be done at the time, but the baby needs to be followed up, and if the testis does not descend it must be brought down surgically at the latest by 5 years of age. If both testes are missing, and in particular if the scrotum is unusually small, consider dysmorphic or intersex problems (p. 318).

HYPOSPADIAS

(p. 320)

CIRCUMCISION

(p. 86)

URINARY TRACT INFECTION

(p. 223)

VAGINAL BLEEDING

A small amount of vaginal bleeding may occur during the first week as an oestrogen withdrawal phenomenon. No treatment is required.

MUCOID VAGINAL DISCHARGE

Many female babies have a small amount of shiny white vaginal discharge during the first week. This is normal, and of no significance.

BABIES NOT PASSING URINE

The paediatrician is frequently summoned to the postnatal ward to see an otherwise normal baby who has never been known to pass urine since birth. This usually means that urine was passed immediately after delivery without being noticed. The baby is often breast-fed and has had a poor fluid intake over the first 24–48 hours. I have never known a baby present in this way with serious illness or malformation. However, to keep everyone happy, I examine the baby and pronounce all is well; one day, who knows, I will find a huge bladder or a baby with Potter's syndrome and normal lungs!

POOR URINARY STREAM

This is a significant piece of history and should always be taken seriously. If there is hypospadias, it probably means meatal stenosis; more seriously it could be the presentation of posterior urethral valves. Neurological bladder problems usually present with some other feature, in particular, neural tube defects. Carefully examine all babies reported to have a poor urinary stream, and unless a good urinary stream appears, and the baby is clinically normal, investigation by urine analysis, renal tract ultrasound and cystography is usually indicated.

LUMPS, BUMPS, TAGS AND HOLES

LYMPHADENOPATHY

In general, lymph nodes are not enlarged in the neonate. If they are, it either suggests congenital infection or is a response to some obvious peripheral infected lesion. Lumps and bumps should, therefore, never be attributed to 'normal' lymph nodes.

NECK LUMPS

Thyroid

A goitre may be found in an area of endemic cretinism, if the mother was taking goitrogens (particularly antithyrotoxicosis medications p. 36), or with various forms of neonatal thyroid disease including neonatal thyrotoxicosis and the inherited defects of thyroxine synthesis. A goitre should always be fully investigated.

A thyroglossal cyst may rarely be found; affected infants may be hypothyroid (p. 115) and the presence of normal thyroid tissue should always be sought by a radioiodine scan.

Branchial cysts

These are fluctuant swellings, usually away from the mid-line, which rarely transilluminate since they are usually full of opalescent fluid. They often have a fistula to a sinus on the neck, and frequently become infected. They should be excised.

Cystic hygroma

These can be small cystic transilluminating swellings in the supraclavicular fossae, or huge multilocular lesions obstructing the airway, and for which urgent tracheostomy may be required immediately after delivery to relieve the airways obstruction. The lesions should always be removed as a planned procedure later in infancy.

Sternomastoid tumour

This is the name given to fusiform swelling found on neonatal examination in the belly of usually just one of the sternomastoid muscles. It is probably a haematoma caused by venous obstruction, oedema and necrosis within the muscle, due to pressure on it during delivery of the anterior shoulder, or the head in a breech presentation, in other words, the same forces that fracture the clavicle and cause an Erb's palsy. As the haematoma and associated muscle damage resolve it may shorten the muscle, pulling the infant's head to one side and causing secondary distortion of his facial growth. Babies with a sternomastoid tumour should be followed up, and if the muscle is becoming tight, should be referred for physiotherapy to stretch it – gently!

LUMPS ON THE HEAD

Most lumps on babies' heads are either cephalhaematomata (p. 249) or odd localised areas where a suture overlap is very prominent. Other lumps are rare, but small encephaloceles or dermoid cysts should always be excluded by skull X-ray supplemented by ultrasound if necessary. Some lumps may be areas of subcutaneous fat necrosis (pp. 282–3) often after a forceps delivery.

PROMINENT XIPHISTERNUM

This structure is often very prominent particularly in babies with diastasis recti (p. 268). The mother can be reassured.

LIPOMATA

These can present in the neonatal period as soft, non-fluctuant, non-transilluminating structures within the subcutaneous tissues. Those close to or over the spine should be viewed with grave suspicion since they often indicate an underlying neural tube defect.

SKIN TAGS

These can occur almost anywhere but are particularly common on or around the face, in the pre-auricular area, and may also be vestigal extra digits on the hands and feet. Unless they have an exceptionally narrow pedicle (when they can be tied off), they should be removed as a formal plastic surgery procedure, otherwise an unsightly scar may result.

BREAST ENGORGEMENT

Enlarged breasts are common in the neonate of both sexes due to the effect of maternal oestrogen. No treatment is required, and the paediatrician should restrain his urge to squeeze them and express a small amount of 'witches milk', though this is often produced spontaneously. Fiddling with the organ increases the likelihood that an abscess will develop. This is characterised by the breast becoming inflamed and tender, in which case antibiotics are indicated.

SACROCOCCYGEAL PIT

Sinuses and dimples anywhere else over the spinal cord must be taken seriously since they usually communicate with the dura (p. 96). However, the very common sacrococcygeal pit which is in the natal cleft *and* distal to the tip of the coccyx never communicates with the dura or even with the filum terminale of the end of the spinal canal. By applying adequate lateral pressure to the buttocks the base of the pit can always be seen.

This pit may be the focus of the lesion that progresses to form a pilonidal sinus later in life. No neonatal treatment is required.

PYREXIAL BABIES

A temperature >37.5°C in a baby on a PNW is usually due to:

- room temperature too high;
- lying in direct sunlight or phototherapy – effectively a radiant heat source;
- over-swaddling the infant, or having his cot near a radiator;
- some combination of all three (common).

These nursing errors should be remedied and if the temperature rapidly falls no further action is required. However, if none of the environmental factors are present, or if the infant looks unwell, or if he is still febrile 60 minutes later, only two conditions should be considered, *infection* (p. 293) and dehydration fever.

DEHYDRATION FEVER

This is usually seen in term infants, often breast-fed, who have lost more than 10 per cent of their birthweight, but who otherwise have no abnormalities on clinical examination. The diagnosis can be confirmed by demonstrating a raised serum osmolality >300 mOsm/kg H_2O. The infant should be given a liberal fluid intake of 10 per cent dextrose if breast-fed, which is usually taken avidly, and restores the temperature to normal over 1–2 hours.

PALLOR

The approach to the very pale baby, acutely ill after delivery, is described on p. 71.

In an otherwise healthy baby pallor usually means anaemia. If the haemoglobin is < 12 g%, then the most likely diagnosis is either a feto-maternal haemorrhage during the delivery (or a twin–twin transfusion, p. 199), bleeding from the cord or placenta during delivery, or merely a baby who missed out on a large part of his placental transfusion at delivery. If the pallor is detected in the first 48–72 hours, it is worth trying to confirm the former diagnosis by examining the mother's blood for fetal RBC (the Kleihauer test).

Another alternative is that the baby has one of the haemolytic disorders which cause neonatal jaundice but his liver is working well and conjugating the bilirubin. Therefore the anaemic baby should also be investigated as outlined on p. 241.

If all these tests are negative, it should be assumed that the neonate did have some unrecognised blood loss in labour, or only a small placental transfusion. If the low haemoglobin is found in the first 24 hours, so long as it is > 10 g/dl, since the haemoglobin concentration normally tends to rise in the first 24–48 hours, no further action is required. However, if after 48 hours it is still < 10 g/dl, he should be given a top-up transfusion of 25 ml/kg of packed cells, and this should also be considered even if his haemoglobin is in the 10–12 g/dl range. Once the haemoglobin is > 12–13 g/dl the baby is safe to go home, though it is probably worthwhile giving him oral iron: 60 mg FeSO o.d. for 1–2 months, and following him up.

The vast majority do well on follow-up, their haemoglobin stays stable, and it can be assumed that their early neonatal anaemia was indeed from one of the disorders outlined above. However, the occasional infant will stay anaemic, and he should be checked for occult blood loss, urinary disease (an important cause of infantile anaemia) or primary red cell or bone marrow disorders.

PLETHORA/POLYCYTHAEMIA

Although polycythaemia is regarded as a serious problem by some neonatologists, I think the diagnosis should only be entertained in babies with symptoms such as fits, dyspnoea or heart failure and a central venous (as opposed to capillary) haematocrit > 70 per cent. Such babies should be on an NNICU. There is no need to screen babies on a PNW for this condition by doing routine haematocrits. However, plethoric babies do have an increased incidence of neonatal jaundice (p. 239), though this does not require any special management beyond that outlined in Chapter 17.

HYPOGLYCAEMIA

There is currently marked controversy about the definition of neonatal hypoglycaemia. As far as normal term babies are concerned the data in Fig. 18.2 would be widely accepted.

The problem comes with pre-term and SFD babies, for whom there is no 'normal' data better than that in Table 18.1. Yet, this was gathered at a time when feeding practice was less enthusiastic than in the 1990s, and may therefore represent abnormally low values. Whether these values are acceptable or not depends on whether being asymptomatic with a blood glucose between 1.0 and 2.5 mmol/l does any harm, and for otherwise well babies there is no such evidence.

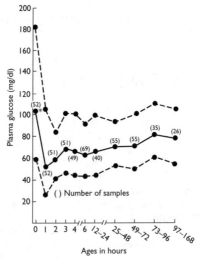

FIGURE 18.2 Predicted plasma glucose values during first week of life in healthy term neonates appropriate for gestational age (from Srinivasan *et al.*, 1986, with permission) (40 mg/dl=2.2 mmol/l)

TABLE 18.1   Blood glucose values for various ages* (mean ± ISD)

Hours				Days					
0–2	2–4	6–12	12–24	1	2	3	4	5	6
41	47	48	45	44	39	40	42	43	43
11.4	12.6	15.8	15.4	12.0	12.8	12.6	11.9	12.2	12.6

*From Cornblath and Schwartz (1976).

While ducking the issue of a definition of hypoglycaemia, I would suggest that:

1 Blood glucose must be kept above 1.0 mmol/l at all times.
2 In sick, pre-term and SFD babies, and infants of diabetic mothers, levels between 1.0 and 2.0 mmol/l in the first 72 hours should be noted, and

dealt with by increasing feeds or the rate of intravenous dextrose. Thereafter levels should be kept
above 2.0 mmol/l.

3 In term babies the level must be kept above 1.5
mmol/l in the first 48 hours and above 2.0 mmol/l
thereafter.

4 If babies over a week old consistently have levels
below 2.5 mmol/l a cause should be sought.

Many babies frequently have blood glucose values
only slightly higher than these lower limits and there
is no evidence at all that this has ever done them any
harm. The neonatal brain can metabolise lactate and
ketones as energy sources, and this probably explains
why many babies tolerate levels even lower than these
cut-off points for hypoglycaemia for several hours
without ever becoming symptomatic (fits or apnoea)
or having any sequelae. This latter feature is very
important to remember when planning routines to
monitor for neonatal hypoglycaemia (p. 185, 211).

Most babies who develop hypoglycaemia as defined
above will either be on the NNICU because they are
ill or < 1.70 kg, or will be included in the screening
programmes outlined in Chapters 11 and 15. The
only other group of normal neonates whom we have
found to develop hypoglycaemia, are breast-fed
babies in whom the feeding is not going well by the
third or fourth day.

If *a*symptomatic hypoglycaemia is detected in any
baby, an immediate feed of 15–20 ml/kg of formula
should be given, and the Dextrostix rechecked
30 minutes later. If it has not risen, the baby
should be admitted to the NNICU for intravenous
dextrose. If it has, the baby should continue in
his previous feeding routine, but if breast-fed
may need to be complemented as outlined on pp.
187–8.

HYPOCALCAEMIA

In the first week of life this is defined as a serum calcium < 1.75 mmol/l (3.5 mEq/l). It is now very rare in an era of breast-feeding and low phosphate cows' milk based formulae, except in ill, low birthweight babies. It is occasionally detected in jittery, small-for-dates, pre-term or diabetic babies, but rarely requires treatment other than giving supplements of calcium gluconate (5–10 ml of 10 per cent calcium gluconate/24 hours) for 2–3 days until the calcium levels rise.

SKIN PROBLEMS

Most babies at birth are covered with a greasy white substance called vernix, the purpose of which is unknown, though it may have an antiseptic purpose.

Many lesions appear on the skin of the normal neonate. Most are harmless and/or birthmarks and treatment is rarely required.

Hair is usually present in a normal distribution on the scalp at birth, but its colour often bears relatively little relationship to that which the baby will achieve in adult life. The more pre-term baby is covered in a very fine generalised downy hair called lanugo which rapidly disappears in the first week after delivery. Occasionally, this hairiness will be more marked, but requires no specific treatment as it usually clears over a longer period of time.

TRAUMA

Friction around the neck, limbs or groin from tight-fitting clothes or nappies may cause local areas of erythema. Fingers and toes may get trapped in clothing causing erythema at the trapped sites, and occasionally peripheral gangrene.

HARLEQUIN COLOUR CHANGE

This is a dramatic, transient (1–2 minutes) colour change with one side of the baby pale and sharply demarcated from the other half which is pink. It rapidly fades and is of no significance.

CUTIS MARMORATA

This is often transient mottling pattern resembling a net seen on the skin of many neonates, particularly if they have been transiently cold. It is entirely normal, and usually disappears when the baby warms up.

MILIA

These are yellow or white spots 1 mm in diameter over the cheeks, nasal bridge and naso-labial folds. They are a normal finding, occur in about 40 per cent of neonates and are small inclusion cysts at the openings of sebaceous glands. No treatment is indicated.

MILIARIA (SWEAT RASH)

These are 1–2 mm superficial non-inflammatory vesicles over the forehead, neck and skin folds; they often burst. They may be induced by a warm environment. No treatment is required other than powdering the affected area.

SUPERNUMARY NIPPLES

A proportion of entirely normal babies have an extra pigmented spot below the normal nipple, on the line that represents the primitive milk ridge of the embryo. Such nipples are never functional and are of no clinical significance.

CONGENITAL ECTODERMAL DEFECTS (APLASIA CUTIS)

Occasionally babies are born with a full thickness skin defect, characteristically 1–2 cm in diameter and over the vertex of the skull. Similar skin defects can occur more rarely in other situations. They are benign and rapidly heal after birth. However, if they occur within the scalp, the scar that forms does not normally get covered with hair.

ERYTHEMA TOXICUM (EOSINOPHIL RASH OF THE NEWBORN)

This maculo-papular rash occurs in 30–70 per cent of normal term neonates (very rare in the pre-term) and although it may be present at birth has a peak incidence at 72–96 hours. It may be mistaken for skin sepsis. The papules appear white or yellow, are full of eosinophils and are surrounded by a flare of erythema. In marked cases the rash may be confluent in some areas. The rash fades by the end of the first week, and no treatment is required.

PUSTULAR MELANOSIS

This rare, benign and transient rash is usually present at birth (unlike toxic erythema). It occurs mainly over the neck, back, forehead and shins and consists of small vesico-pustules that rupture within 24–48 hours, leaving a central hyperpigmented macule with a collar of scale. The vesicles contain polymorphs and are sterile, and the macules may persist for a few months. The condition should be differentiated from infection, and does not require treatment.

SUBCUTANEOUS FAT NECROSIS

This is usually seen in areas of skin that have had pressure applied to them, e.g. by forceps blades (p. 250) or by the pelvis during labour. It consists of firm raised reddish purple lesions up to 1 cm in diameter which feel as though they involve the full thickness of the skin and subcutaneous tissue. Histologically, as the name implies, there is fat necrosis and sometimes calcification in the tissue. No treatment is required, and the lesions resolve fully, though this may take 4–6 weeks.

NAPPY RASH

In the neonatal period this common rash is usually perianal and caused by friction or irritation from faeces. It generally responds to barrier creams or exposure. Monilial nappy rash is described on pp. 222–3. The more traditional ammoniacal nappy rash on the upper thighs and abdomen as well as in the perineal area usually develops after the baby has left the maternity hospital. It responds to barrier creams, clean or disposable nappies, and if severe, exposure.

SEBORRHOEIC DERMATITIS

This is rare in the neonate, apart from a small amount of weeping erythema in the skin creases and groin. After the neonatal period, when it may become severe, it is usually associated with thick greasy scales on the scalp (cradle cap) and a severe seborrhoeic nappy rash. Treatment is with exposure, removing the cradle cap with a keratolytic ointment, and by topical steroids.

SKIN INFECTION

(p. 222)

PETECHIAL SKIN RASHES

Petechiae, if generalised, usually signify thrombocytopenia. In a well infant this may be autoimmune (p. 28) or isoimmune. In an ill infant it strongly suggests infection, either congenital or acquired. After confirming thrombocytopenia by platelet count, further investigation is always indicated.

NAEVI AND BIRTHMARKS

In general these are benign, but any form of naevus, haemangiomatous or melanomatous, which occurs over the line of the spine below the area of the nape naevus must always be viewed with suspicion as it may be a marker of some underlying abnormality of the spinal cord.

Mongolian spots

These are found in 90 per cent of coloured or oriental children and consist of grey-blue pigmented areas, 2–10 cm in diameter, chiefly over the buttocks, flanks and shoulders. They are much rarer in Caucasians.

The simple naevus (Salmon patch, 'stork bite')

This is the most common capillary haemangioma type of birthmark, and occurs on the root of the nose and on to the forehead, on the eyelids, and at the nape of the neck. They all fade to some extent during childhood, but the nape naevi are common in adult life, and the others may flare up when an adult is embarrassed.

Port wine stain (naevus flammeus)

These permanent, sharply circumscribed, reddish purple lesions can occur anywhere on the body but are common over the face. They do not fade. Those lying over the trigeminal area may be associated with ipsilateral intracranial haemangioimata (Sturge-Weber syndrome) often with convulsions, hemiparesis and mental retardation.

Strawberry naevi

These start as small bright red macules noted at birth which gradually enlarge over the next 6–9 months to form a raised strawberry. They can occur anywhere in the body, are often multiple, and begin to regress at the end of the first year. They disappear virtually completely, and only need treatment if they cause problems round the eyes, mouth or perineum. Multiple ones occasionally cause heart failure.

Cavernous haemangioma

These lesions lie deeper in the dermis and are less well defined than the strawberry. They give a bluish discolouration to the overlying skin and may feel like a 'bag of worms'. Sometimes there are mixed strawberry and cavernous lesions. Although they may partially involute, they rarely disappear completely.

Melanotic naevi

A wide selection of brown birthmarks are present at birth. The vast majority of these are entirely harmless, and need no treatment at all. The rare giant hairy naevus with a deeply pigmented lesion may be extensive. This is one of the few naevi which require early treatment, because they may turn malignant.

EPIDERMOLYSIS BULLOSA

This is the most common inherited skin disease in the neonate. Blisters may be present at birth, and commonly appear at sites of friction thereafter. There are many variants of the disease, and management depends on the differential diagnosis on the basis of the clinical pattern of the disease and skin biopsy.

LIMB ABNORMALITIES

These are described on p. 318.

REFERENCES

Cornblath, M. and Schwartz, R. (1976). *Disorders of Carbohydrate Metabolism in Infancy*. 2nd Ed. W.B. Saunders, Philadelphia, pp. 78–79.

Hensinger, R.N. and Jones, R.T. (1992). Orthopaedic problems in the newborn. In: *Textbook of Neonatology*, 2nd Edn Ed. Roberton N.R.C. pp. 899–914.

Lilien, L.D., Srinivasan, G., Pyati, S.P., Yeh, T.F. and Piles, R.S. (1986). Green vomiting in the first 72 hours in normal infants. *American Journal of Diseases of Children* **140**, 662–664.

Srinivasan, G., Pildes, R.S., Cattamachi, G., Voora, S. and Lilien, L.D. (1986). Plasma glucose values in normal neonates. *Journal of Pediatrics* **109**, 114–117.

19

SERIOUS ILLNESS PRESENTING IN A PREVIOUSLY WELL NEONATE

———

The conditions described in this chapter are those which may come on, usually in the first day or two after delivery, and which require urgent transfer to the NNICU whether the baby is at home or on the PNW.

RESPIRATORY PROBLEMS

TACHYPNOEA, DYSPNOEA <6 HOURS OF AGE

Within the first 4–6 hours of life any infant who was well in the labour ward may develop signs of respiratory distress. This is more likely to be the case in the pre-term infants described in Chapter 11. The classical triad of respiratory illness presenting in the first 4–6 hours is tachypnoea >60/min, dyspnoea (intercostal/subcostal recession, flaring nostrils, sternal retraction) and an expiratory grunt. Respiratory distress at this time can be due to any of the conditions listed in Table 19.1. However, the most likely are mild RDS, transient tachypnoea of the newborn (TTN), a small pneumothorax or a pneumomediastinum, and most important of all pneumonia with or without septicaemia. All dyspnoeic neonates must have a chest X-ray, be worked up for infection

TABLE 19.1 Causes of early onset dyspnoea

- Respiratory distress syndrome
- Meconium aspiration
- Birth asphyxia and acidaemia
- Transient tachypnoea of the newborn
- Pneumonia (especially group B streptococcal)
- Pneumothorax, pneumomediastinum
- Persistent fetal circulation
- Congenital defects
    Congenital heart disease with heart failure
    Diaphragmatic hernia
    Lung malformation

(p. 298) and transferred to an NNICU. Early onset infection can disseminate very rapidly in such infants, so if there is likely to be delay in transferring the baby to an NNICU, after taking a blood culture start him on penicillin (50 000u/ kg/dose) and gentamicin 2.5 mg/kg/dose.

RESPIRATORY ILLNESS >6 HOURS OF AGE

A baby may also present after 6 hours of age with the classical triad of respiratory illness (see above). There are only two likely diagnoses in such babies: heart failure (see below, and p. 261) and pneumonia. Differentiating between these two possibilities is usually very easy on the basis of clinical examination, a CXR and an echocardiogram. If infection seems likely, the baby must have a full infectious disease work-up, and if there is likely to be a delay in transferring him to an NNICU start penicillin and gentamicin; if he is > 48 hours old substitute flucloxacillin 30 mg/kg/dose for the penicillin.

APNOEIC ATTACK/CHOKING ATTACK

(see also tracheo-oesophageal fistula, p.290)

A not uncommon story is that a previously normal baby, usually during or just after a feed, chokes or splutters, goes transiently blue, makes a rapid recovery with or without some oropharyngeal suction but is often a bit pale and floppy for 30–60 minutes afterwards. It is probably worth admitting such babies to the NNICU for observation and a CXR to exclude aspiration pneumonia. However, precious little usually comes of such attacks, the baby behaves and feeds impeccably after NNICU admission, and can usually be returned to his mother on the PNW 24–48 hours later.

Genuine apnoeic attacks are much more of a problem for sick VLBW neonates in a NNICU, but are rare in the babies described in this book. However, if a baby does have one on a PNW, it may be a sequel of birth asphyxia or respiratory depression from the drugs administered to the mother in labour. Other causes include infection, a convulsion and metabolic problems especially hypoglycaemia (p. 277).

Treatment

If a baby is found apnoeic, his resuscitation is exactly the same as that described in Chapter 4 for a baby apnoeic after delivery (pp. 65–6). The baby on a postnatal ward who has had an apnoeic attack has, of course, been breathing satisfactorily for some time, and this makes resuscitation easier. Always aspirate his nose and mouth in case there is any milk or vomit there. Peripheral stimuli, e.g. flicking his feet will often evoke a cry, and if this does not work he will virtually always respond to bag and mask resuscitation (p. 64). For the babies on a postnatal ward who are > 32 weeks gestation and therefore not at risk from retinopathy of prematurity, it is safe in the short term to administer a high oxygen concentration by the bag and mask during resuscitation.

Once such a baby is breathing satisfactorily, he should be admitted to the NNICU for diagnostic work-up, monitoring and appropriate therapy.

SUDDEN INFANT DEATH SYNDROME (SIDS)

True SIDS can and does occur in the first week. As with all SIDS, nothing can be done to anticipate it, or to prevent it.

STRIDOR

(p. 259)

TRACHEO-OESOPHAGEAL FISTULA

Babies with this condition should be diagnosed within the first 3–4 hours of life on the basis of:

- The history of maternal polyhydramnios, because the fetus cannot swallow.
- Early postnatal problems with swallowing. The baby is always spluttering and choking, and cannot swallow his secretions.

In a baby with these symptoms the diagnosis of TOF is made by trying to pass a wide-bore (FG8) or naso-gastric tube. Do not use a fine NG tube since this curls up in the upper oesophageal pouch and gives a false impression of how far in the tube has gone. If a wide-bore tube cannot be inserted, confirm the diagnosis by taking a plain CXR which will show the tube held up at the T1–T2 level. Leave this tube in situ and aspirate it continuously while transferring the baby for surgery. The sooner this is done the better.

CARDIOVASCULAR PROBLEMS

CYANOSIS

Paediatricians are often summoned to a PNW to see a baby who is blue. Usually the diagnosis is either trau-matic facial cyanosis (p. 251) or the peripheral and perioral blueness which is a very common finding in entirely normal babies. However, if genuine central cyanosis is present, this usually means heart disease.

Pulmonary disease usually presents on a PNW with the signs of respiratory distress, and not with cyanosis which is a sign of severe pulmonary disease, and would suggest that the early signs of the illness must have been present and not recognised for hours if not days.

Therefore a baby who is found to be genuinely cyanosed on a PNW can be assumed to be suffering from cyanotic congenital heart disease until proved otherwise. He needs a CXR, ECG, echocardiogram and transfer to a regional neonatal cardiac unit as soon as possible. Always discuss the patient with this unit pre-transfer so that appropriate treatment with diuretics, digoxin or prostaglandin E can be started immediately.

HEART FAILURE

The signs of heart failure in a neonate are given on p. 261. Hopefully the neonate on a PNW will present with the early features such as poor feeding, tachypnoea and mild tachycardia.

By the time a neonate is in heart failure, in addition to some enlargement of the liver and spleen and perhaps some crepitations in the lungs if there is left ventricular failure, murmurs are usually present, unless the failure is due to primary myocardial disease such as myocarditis or fibroelastosis. Coarctation is one of the common causes of heart failure in the first week, and so the femoral pulses and leg blood pressure must always be checked. Cyanosis may coexist if the heart failure is due to a cyanotic form of CHD.

The infant should be admitted to the NNICU, investigated by a CXR, ECG and echocardiogram, and his heart failure treated by fluid restriction, diuretics and oxygen. In general babies who develop heart failure in the first week have major defects and they should be referred to the regional neonatal cardiac unit for assessment (see above).

NEUROLOGICAL PROBLEMS

Meningomyelocoele is described on p. 321; hypertonia and hypotonia on pp. 255–7. If the baby suddenly becomes hypotonic and listless, as well as sepsis (p. 295), always remember the inherited organic acidaemias and hyperammonaemias (Table 19.2), all of which require urgent transfer to a neonatal unit.

TABLE 19.2 Rare metabolic errors presenting in the neonatal period with neurological symptoms, apnoea or hyperventilation

- Maple syrup urine disease
- Isovaleric acidaemia
- Propionicacidaemia
- Multiple carboxylase deficiency
- Methylmalonic acidaemia
- Non-ketotic hyperglycinaemia (glycine encephalopathy)
- Primary lactic acidosis
- Ornithine transcarbamylase deficiency
- Argininosuccinic aciduria
- Citrullinaemia
- Carbamyl phosphate synthetase deficiency
- Hyperargininaemia

CONVULSIONS

A common problem with babies who develop fits on a postnatal ward is that only the mother sees them. However, one of the first rules of neonatology, is that if a mother thinks her baby has had a fit, she should be believed. Get her to mimic what she saw and remember that the physical manifestations of a seizure in a neonate can be very subtle. Unless the mother clearly describes jitteriness (p. 258) or the single myoclonic jerk that babies often have as they drop off to sleep, the baby should be admitted to the NNICU, and put in an incubator where he can be carefully observed. Since there are multiple causes for neonatal fits, the only safe approach is to do all the tests listed in Table 19.3 as an initial work-up. If

TABLE 19.3 Routine investigation of a neonate with convulsions

- Blood glucose
- Electrolytes and blood urea
- Calcium
- WBC and differential blood culture
- Blood culture
- Lumbar puncture
- Ultrasound brain scan

they are all negative, but fits continue, further biochemical investigation for an inborn error metabolism, EEG and CT scan, is indicated.

SERIOUS INFECTION

This is probably the most common, important and potentially fatal condition which can develop in a previously asymptomatic baby on a postnatal ward or at home, and recognising the problem early is of crucial importance since the comparative immunodeficiency of the neonate (p. 217) not only predisposes him to the infection, but means that when infection occurs it may disseminate very rapidly with septicaemic shock and death occurring within 12 hours of the first signs of illness. This has two major implications:

- Early diagnosis is essential. Even very trivial clinical findings suggesting infection demand full laboratory evaluation.
- Initial therapy must be started on the basis of clinical suspicion. There is no time to wait for the laboratory results to come back 24–48 hours later.

The two cornerstones of early diagnosis are always taking seriously any anxieties a mother has about her baby, coupled with shrewd, experienced and vigilant routine observations of the baby by the nurses. Woe betide the doctor who ignores such clinical leads.

ORGANISMS

It behoves every paediatrician to know the organisms responsible for most of the infections developing in babies in his maternity hospital, and also to know which antibiotics they are likely to be sensitive to. For infections presenting on a PNW, the likely pathogens in Britain are group B streptococci, staphylococci and *E. coli*, sensitive to, respectively, penicillin, flucloxacillin and aminoglycosides, but many other organisms can be responsible.

TYPE OF INFECTION

Serious infection, e.g. pneumonia and meningitis in the neonate is virtually always accompanied by a septicaemia. Given that babies with septicaemia without pneumonia frequently have apnoeic attacks or tachypnoea, and that signs of meningism are absent in neonatal meningitis, it can be understood why the history and clinical features of all types of serious infection in the neonate are surprisingly uniform, and why in the early stages of the illness they will rarely give a clue as to the primary site of infection (see below).

HISTORY

Apart from verifying the presenting history, the following points should always be checked:
• Was there anything in the perinatal history suggesting an infectious risk, e.g. maternal illness or pyrexia, prolonged rupture of membranes, pathogens present in the maternal HVS?
• Is there a risk of nosocomial infection from relatives, staff or other sick infants in the ward?

CLINICAL FEATURES (EARLY)

The early symptoms and signs are virtually always non-specific, but the aim of every neonatal service should be to recognise all infections at this stage rather than wait until organ-specific features develop (v.i.).

Temperature change

Hypothermia and hyperthermia are often due to deficiencies in the control of the environmental temperature (pp. 74, 275). These can usually be excluded rapidly by taking a history, and noting the environmental temperature! A body temperature < 36°C or > 37.5°C sustained for more than an hour or two in an appropriate environmental temperature is, however, due to infection until proved otherwise. The higher or lower the temperature, the more significant it is.

Anorexia

When a previously healthy baby refuses to feed from breast or bottle, infection should be suspected.

Poor weight gain

This, without any other symptoms can indicate occult infection, though it is obviously not a feature of rapidly progressing sepsis.

Listlessness, lethargy, hypotonia, pallor, mottled skin

These are often the first, mild, non-specific signs that a baby is unwell. The baby just does not seem 'right'.

Irritability

A baby who is irritable and will not stop crying or whimpering even for a feed may be developing septicaemia or meningitis.

Jaundice

If this develops rapidly in a baby without haemolytic disease, sepsis is present until proved otherwise.

Vomiting

If persistent, this is suggestive of infection (as well as intestinal obstruction). Diarrhoea and vomiting are not necessarily signs of gastroenteritis in neonates, and are much more commonly non-specific features of early infection.

Ileus/intestinal obstruction

Sepsis may present as vomiting, abdominal distension and constipation due to an ileus, particularly when there is intra-abdominal infection, e.g. necrotising enterocolitis (p. 301).

Pseudoparalysis

The lack of movement due to limb pain may alert the clinician to the presence of arthritis or osteomyelitis before local or generalised signs develop.

Apnoea

Commonly the first signs of infection in premature infants, including those of 32–35 weeks gestation on a postnatal ward.

Tachypnoea

Tachypnoea accompanying any of the above signs is often the first sign of pneumonia or septicaemia.

Cardiovascular

Tachycardia is common in infection especially cardiac infections. Delayed capillary filling after blanching the skin may also suggest infection.

CLINICAL FEATURES (LATE)

These are usually specific to one organ system, and if infection presents in this way it suggests that the diagnosis could have been made earlier if the infant had been more carefully and expertly observed.

• **Respiratory**:	Cyanosis, grunting, respiratory distress, cough.
• **Abdominal**:	Bilious or faeculent vomiting, gross abdominal distension, livid flanks and periumbilical staining, absent bowel sounds.

• **CNS**:	High pitched cry, retracted head, bulging fontanelle, convulsion.
• **Haemorrhagic diathesis**:	Petechiae. Bleeding from puncture sites.
• **Sclerema**:	This is a late non-specific sign of any serious illness, including infection.

EXAMINATION

The baby should be completely undressed and carefully examined, paying particular attention to the following points:

- Confirming the presenting signs, e.g. fever, jaundice, pallor, grunting.
- Are there any lesions on the skin, subcutaneous tissues or scalp?
- Is there periodic breathing or tachypnoea at rest?
- Is there a tachycardia or murmurs?
- Are there added sounds on auscultation of the chest?
- Is there hepatosplenomegaly which accompanies generalised infection as well as hepatitis?
- Is there kidney enlargement, since cortical swelling of the kidneys may be present in early septicaemia as well as UTI?
- Is the umbilicus red and tender with a thickened cord of inflamed umbilical vein extending up the falciform ligament?
- Can oesteomyelitis and arthritis be excluded by the presence of full and painless limb movements?
- Are bowel sounds present; does the infant cry during palpation of his abdomen suggesting peritonitis?
- Do not forget otitis media in the neonate.
- Meningism is rare in neonatal meningitis, but check the spinal cord, column and skull for pits or other skin defects that might be the entry site for

spinal infection.
- Is there any evidence of an altered neurological state, e.g. coma?
- Infants do not have dysuria or frequency, but with pyelonephritis they may have loin tenderness which can be detected by a gentle pressure on the renal angle.
- Is the infant dehydrated; has he lost more than 10 per cent of his birthweight suggesting major gut fluid loss?

INVESTIGATION

Full investigation of a baby with a strong suspicion of septicaemia should take place in the neonatal unit, the tests needed include:
- a throat swab and swabs of any skin lesions;
- external ear swabs can be taken in the first 12 hours of life;
- stool culture or effective rectal swab (only in babies with diarrhoea);
- bag urine;
- blood culture;
- WBC and differential;
- CRP;
- chest X-ray;
- blood gases;
- lumbar puncture;
- antigen detection tests, e.g. latex tests, if available.

Some of these can be carried out immediately, particularly if there is likely to be delay in the infant being transferred to a neonatal intensive care unit. After consultation with that unit, and taking a blood culture, it may be justifiable to start an intravenous infusion and administer antibiotics, the usual cocktail being penicillin/flucloxacillin plus gentamicin (p. 285).

GASTROINTESTINAL PROBLEMS

GASTROENTERITIS

(p. 225)

ABDOMINAL DISTENSION

Abdominal distension may be due to enlargement of the liver, spleen, bladder or kidneys above the normal range (Chapter 7). Which one is enlarged is usually obvious on clinical examination, and abdominal ultrasound will confirm the diagnosis. Intra-abdominal tumours may also present in the neonatal period. The differential diagnosis of enlargement of the viscera is given in Table 19.4; appropriate investigations are usually easy to carry out.

TABLE 19.4 Differential diagnosis of enlarged abdominal organs in the neonate

Liver/spleen	Blood group incompatibility
	Heart failure
	Hepatitis/congenital or acquired; infection
	Generalised sepsis
	Rarities – tumours, haematological malignancy, inborn metabolic errors
Kidney	Hydronephrosis
	Cystic dysplasia
	Polycystic
	Renal vein thrombosis
Bladder	Posterior urethral valves
	Retention of urine from any cause

If the abdomen is distended but no masses can be felt, or the abdomen is so rigid that it is impossible to palpate, this could have six causes.
- Fluid/ascites – including a urinary leak; rarely blood.
- Pneumoperitoneum – leak from the chest or a ruptured viscus.

- Peritonitis with guarding and rigidity.
- Congenital absence of the abdominal muscles –
  prune-belly syndrome and variants.
- Intestinal obstruction
    with bowel inflammation
    congenital, structural.
- Normal big belly.

Clinical examination, combined with plain abdominal X-ray and ultrasound will rapidly establish the differential after the baby has been transferred to the NNICU.

INTESTINAL OBSTRUCTION

In general, the features of significant obstruction are copious, usually bilious vomiting, abdominal distension and failure to pass meconium, though babies with high obstruction such as duodenal or jejunal atresia may often pass one or two lots of meconium. A diagnosis must be established as expeditiously as possible since in one cause of neonatal obstruction, a volvulus of a malrotation, if the diagnosis is delayed a large part of the small intestine may be infarcted, whereas if the diagnosis is made early the volvulus can be untwisted at laparotomy while the bowel is still viable. In general, clinical examination has comparatively little to offer in the baby with intestinal obstruction except for the following:

- Is there an anus, and is it in the right position?
- Rectal examination – though this should be avoided if the putative diagnosis is Hirschsprung's since by provoking the release of stool it makes radiological diagnosis difficult.
- Palpable faecal masses are very suggestive of meconium ileus (neonatal cystic fibrosis).
- Are there any signs of intra-abdominal inflammation (redness, tenderness) suggesting necrotising enterocolitis?
- Absent bowel sounds are always an ominous sign of intra-abdominal inflammation.

A baby suspected of obstruction must be investigated at once by plain abdominal X-ray and appropriate contrast studies, proceeding urgently to laparotomy if indicated.

NECROTISING ENTEROCOLITIS

Although this is much more common in pre-term infants, epidemics as well as sporadic cases can occur in previously normal, full term infants on a PNW. They usually present as ill, septic babies with a distended, often tender abdomen and bloody stools. The diagnosis is confirmed by seeing pneumatosis intestinalis on a plain X-ray of the abdomen.

HAEMORRHAGE

Most pale babies are either asphyxiated or have bled intrapartum (p. 71). Most babies who present with haematemesis or melaena are not acutely ill and the blood 'lost' is often ingested maternal blood (pp. 264–5).

However, if a baby is genuinely thought to have bled, and the blood lost from any site (bowel, umbilicus etc.) is proven neonatal on Apt's test (p.264), it is essential to admit the baby to the NNICU for assessment. One of the real problems is that midwives used to the labour ward may not be impressed by the spilling of 100 ml of blood and may seriously underestimate the significance of such a bleed in a baby in whom it may represent 50 per cent of his blood volume. As with all acute haemorrhages, the patient may initially sustain his blood pressure and PCV, but useful early signs of a big neonatal haemorrhage are tachypnoea, tachycardia and a metabolic acidaemia. Major postnatal (as apposed to intrapartum) haemorrhage usually occurs only when a cord ligature or clamp falls off, or from the GI tract or umbilical stump (and at the risk of boring readers by repeating myself yet again) in hospitals where universal vitamin K prophylaxis has been abandoned.

Rare causes of major neonatal haemorrhage are subgaleal haemorrhage (p. 250), haemorrage following circumcision in a haemophiliac (or a baby not given vitamin K), or intra-abdominal haemorrhage from a ruptured viscus (though these babies have usually suffered severe intrapartum trauma and are already on the NNICU). Haemorrhage from a Meckel's diverticulum is extremely rare in the neonate.

SUDDEN COLLAPSE

There are very few things that can suddenly cause a term baby, thought to be well 2–3 hours before, suddenly to appear very ill. These include:

- overwhelming sepsis;
- congenital heart disease;
- intracranial haemorrhage;
- systemic haemorrhage;
- addisonian crisis;
- inborn error of metabolism;
- fits.

OVERWHELMING SEPSIS

This usually occurs in the first 24–48 hours when infection was acquired intrapartum. After this age, it can happen particularly if the baby develops meningitis, severe NEC or one of the rapidly progressive viraemias, e.g. herpes, coxsackie or Echo. Diagnostic clues localising the infection to one system or the other are usually present, and in any case come to light with the infectious disease work-up (p. 298).

CONGENITAL HEART DISEASE

Babies with two forms of congenital heart disease, hypoplastic left heart, and interrupted aortic arch or aortic atresia (which are both variants of the same condition), often do surprisingly well for 48 hours or so and then, when the ductus closes, suddenly collapse with cyanosis, low output and gross heart failure. ECG, CXR and, in particular, echocardiography establish the diagnosis. Urgent referral to the regional cardiac unit is indicated unless the condition is inoperable as with hypoplastic left heart.

INTRACRANIAL HAEMORRHAGE

Even in the mature baby who is not asphyxiated at birth a sudden intracranial haemorrhage can occasionally occur. The baby not only becomes acutely ill, but has symptoms suggesting a CNS problem. The diagnosis can then usually be established easily by cranial ultrasound.

HAEMORRHAGE

(v.s.)

ADDISONIAN CRISIS

Any male infant who suddenly collapses with vomiting, pallor or hypotension in the first 10 days of life should be suspected of having congenital adrenal hyperplasia (p. 319), especially if his nipples, scrotum or penis appear to be too pigmented. The female infant rarely presents this way unless the genital ambiguity (p. 318) was missed at birth.

The infant will usually have hyponatremia and hyperkalaemia, and is often profoundly hypoglycaemic. He should be resuscitated with intravenous glucose, normal saline, and 50 mg of i.v. hydrocortisone; appropriate investigations should be done (p. 319).

INBORN ERRORS OF METABOLISM

The babies with the conditions listed on Table 19.2 usually deteriorate over a period of several hours, but this diagnosis should always be considered in a floppy baby who is hyperventilating and having fits, in particular if there is a family history of previous unexplained neonatal death.

CONVULSIONS

A baby found just after a fit may look dreadful, though quickly perks up as the fit passes. This scenario should be recognised for what it is, and the neonate investigated appropriately (p. 293).

20

MALFORMATIONS

―

ANTENATALLY DIAGNOSED STRUCTURAL MALFORMATIONS

An increasing number of structural malformations are now being identified on antenatal ultrasound. The first thing to say on the topic is that this procedure is not uniformly accurate. Lesions may be missed. This is particularly important where cardiovascular defects are concerned. Antenatal echocardiography will not defect many conditions including the milder/smaller versions of VSD, ASD, coarctation, pulmonary stenosis and aortic stenosis – i.e. all the common forms of congenital heart disease.

Perhaps more importantly, however, lesions identified in utero may not be found after delivery, either because the antenatal diagnosis is wrong or because the lesion has regressed. Therefore, be prepared for a surprise when the baby is born; either he is much better or much worse than anticipated. The parents in this situation often need very careful advice. They may find it surprisingly difficult to form a happy relationship with an entirely normal baby when for the last few weeks or months of the pregnancy they had been anticipating a profoundly abnormal one.

POSTNATAL MANAGEMENT

With malformations like meningomyelocele, diaphragmatic hernia or exomphalos, admission to the neonatal unit and urgent surgery is mandatory. However, with other disorders a more conservative approach can be taken with the baby being admitted to the PNW with his mother and investigated from there.

Renal disorders

These are the most common lesions in which an antenatal diagnosis of a potentially serious condition is combined with a well-grown asymptomatic apparently normal neonate. The conditions identified the most often antenatally are hydronephrosis with pelviureteric junction (PUJ) obstruction, vesicoureteric junction (VUJ) obstruction, multicystic dysplastic kidneys (MCD) and vesicoureteric reflux (VUR). Other disorders found antenatally include posterior urethal valves and a wide variety of structural malformations of the renal tract. Although different urologists and nephrologists vary in their work-up of the baby after birth, the protocol outlined in Fig. 20.1 would be common to many units.

Soft tissue abnormalities

With conditions like cystic hygroma and skeletal defects, nothing is usually required postnatally other than confirmation of the diagnosis by X-ray or CT scan. Giant cystic hygromas may compromise the airway and require NNICU admission.

Intrathoracic lesions

Some babies with intrathoracic masses are asymptomatic when born. If they remain so over the next hour or so, a plain CXR will establish whether the antenatally diagnosed lesion is still present and what size it is. If it is small and seems unlikely to compromise respiration, the baby can be admitted to the PNW with his mother, and further imaging to establish the diagnosis carried out as quickly as possible.

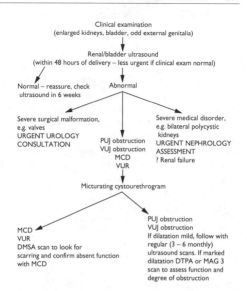

FIGURE 20.1 Evaluation of baby with antenatal diagnosis of renal defect.

Intra-abdominal lesions

The most common intra-abdominal abnormalities are those of the renal tract (v.s.).

Enlargement of the liver and spleen will need appropriate evaluation for haematological, infectious, storage or even malignant conditions, and the latter, particularly neuroblastoma, should be considered for intra-abdominal and retroperitoneal masses. Dilated loops of bowel antenatally may indicate a condition likely to cause intestinal obstruction postnatally.

Gynaecological disorders

Hydrocolpos and its variants may be detected antenatally and will need full evaluation after delivery. Ovarian cysts commonly involute postnatally, but this should be checked by serial ultrasound. Only if their size is causing a clinical problem should they be removed.

CNS disorders

A wide variety of structural malformations of the brain may be detected during routine antenatal ultrasound with BPD measurements. The baby often appears normal at birth but the presence or absence of the defect must be confirmed as soon after delivery as possible by ultrasound, CT or MR scan. The common antenatally detected condition of choroid plexus cysts is benign and does not require further evaluation in the clinically normal baby.

POSTNATALLY DIAGNOSED MALFORMATIONS

Many of the malformations which are apparent immediately after birth, even quite horrific ones like bilateral harelip and cleft palate, major limb reduction defects or Down's syndrome do not actually pose any immediate threat to health, and so the baby does not need admission to the neonatal unit. Nor is it in the mother's interest to keep the baby away from her, since her conceptions of her malformed baby, if she is not allowed to see him, are inevitably much worse than the reality (Drostar *et al.*, 1975). Furthermore, since he will survive, she needs to start to learn as soon as possible any specialised techniques which will be necessary for his long-term care (such as feeding a baby with a cleft palate), and the sooner this gets under way the better. This chapter, therefore deals with the management of those malformations which can and should be cared for on a postnatal ward, most of the care being given by the babies' mothers.

DYSMORPHIC SYNDROMES

Paediatricians are often asked to check out a baby who is thought to look odd. In addition, of course, to doing a full clinical examination, always examine such babies carefully for the many small features that go with dysmorphic syndromes (Table 20.1).

TABLE 20.1 Clinical findings which should alert the clinician to the presence of a dysmorphic syndrome

Odd facial appearance	Small-for-dates
Microcephaly	Abnormal tongue
Big-head, hydrocephalus	Thick gums
Odd shaped head	Receding mandible
Wide fontanelles	Small, low set, simple ears
Coloboma	Neck short or webbed
Cataract	Polydactyly
Microphthalmia	Clinodactyly

In most situations, the conclusion is that he is a normal baby, particularly after looking at one or both his parents whom he resembles. If this is not the conclusion, then he should be checked in the syndrome catalogue books (Jones, 1988), or against one of the computerised syndrome diagnostic systems such as the one produced by the Institute of Child Health in London. A karyotype must always be done in any baby who is considered to be dysmorphic. If his karyotype is normal, and his phenotype cannot be found in any of the catalogues or computer programs, and the abnormalities are few and minor, the parents should be given a good prognosis for subsequent neurological development. The more malformations there are, and the bigger they are, then the more guarded should be the developmental prognosis. It is usually wise to refer such babies, and those in whom a definite diagnosis is made, for genetic counselling.

DOWN'S SYNDROME

This is the most common dysmorphic syndrome. Ninety-five per cent of the patients with the condition have trisomy of chromosome 21. Of the other 5 per cent, a half have translocations and the other half are mosaics. The incidence of trisomy 21 increases with increasing maternal age. Women who become pregnant over the age of 35, and in particular those aged over 40, should have antenatal diagnosis early in the 2nd trimester to exclude this and other rarer chromosomal abnormalities associated with increasing parental age. However since most babies are born to women who are under 35, despite the much lower incidence of Down's syndrome in such women, most Down's babies have young mothers.

The characteristic features of Down's syndrome are listed in Table 20.2. In my experience in recent years, the diagnosis is usually made by an alert midwife either in the labour ward or on the postnatal ward. It is then usually possible for the paediatrician to stage manage a visit to the postnatal ward nursery to examine the baby out of sight of the parents and to confirm the diagnosis clinically, although many parents have in any case already spotted the diagnosis themselves. It is rarely if ever necessary to do a karyotype to confirm the diagnosis; a karyotype should, nevertheless, always be done since if it shows a translocation, although this makes no difference to the baby himself, it does have very different genetic implications for the parents for whom the chance of recurrence may be 1:4 or 5 or worse. Some infants with Down's syndrome have serious heart and gut malformations (Table 20.2); if these are present the infant will, of course, need to be admitted to the NNICU where each problem should be treated on its merits. In the absence of these conditions the neonate with Down's syndrome should stay with his mother on a postnatal ward so she can learn to care

TABLE 20.2 Clinical features of Down's syndrome in the neonatal period

- Small-for-dates
- Hypotonia
- Flat occiput
- 3rd fontanelle
- Microcephaly
- Upward slanting eyes
- Epicanthus
- Brushfield's spots
- Low set, simple ears
- Small nose
- Fissured protruding tongue
- Short hands
- Single palmar crease
- Clinodactyly 5th finger
- Distal palmar triradius
- Gap between first and second toes
- Diastasis recti
- Serious structural defects:
  duodenal atresia
  tracheo-oesphageal fistula
  Hirschsprung's disease
  Congenital heart disease

for him. In fact, the care of a neonatal Down's baby is no different from that of a normal baby since they usually feed well and pose no other problems.

Telling the parents

There are only two rules in this situation, one absolute and one near to absolute. The absolute rule is never lie. Nurses and junior medical staff can evade and pass the buck to the senior paediatric staff, but should never say the baby is fine. The near absolute rule is that the parents should be told before the child leaves the hospital. I have never *not* done this, and I find it difficult to conceive a situation in which it would be better to let the parents get to know their baby as 'normal' only to tell them later that he has Down's syndrome when they would clearly realise that information had been kept from them hitherto.

In general try to see the parents together and have the baby there as well; having a senior nurse from the PNW or NNICU present is also often helpful. The interview should be done in private, not in an open ward. There is no nice way of giving bad news; all that one can do, is to do it sympathetically. Parents remember how they were told, rather than where, when and what. It is I believe, useful at this stage to emphasise the good points of their baby and how normally he is behaving. After a brief optimistic outline of what Down's syndrome babies can do, I leave the parents to themselves; they are usually in no state to take in the details of the long-term management of their handicapped baby. It is necessary to cover these points with the parents in repeated visits over the next few days. The parents may find it helpful to be visited by a local representative of the Down's Syndrome Association.

The criteria for discharging babies with Down's syndrome are no different from those for any other baby. Suitable follow-up arrangements with the local child development clinic should be arranged.

HARELIP, CLEFT PALATE, MID-LINE CLEFT PALATE

Most babies with these malformations should be nursed on a PNW with their mothers who are going to have to learn to feed them for several months until the palate is repaired, and the sooner they start to learn the better. Babies with Pierre Robin syndrome (mid-line cleft, mandibular hypoplasia and glossoptosis) have frequent and severe airways problems and need to be on a NNICU.

The defect of harelip and cleft palate does look gruesome, and of course is immediately apparent to the parents who should be counselled as soon as possible with 'before and after' photographs demonstrating the excellent cosmetic results from surgery.

Always aim to feed the baby normally. In those with just a harelip but no, or minimal, palate defect there are rarely any problems. In those with palatal defects, in general the bigger the defect, the more likely it is that there will be problems. These may be avoided by using a dental palatal prosthesis which closes off the defect, and gives the baby something to press the nipple against with his tongue and lower jaw.

With a little practice, the feeding usually goes very well. In bottle-fed babies a large hole in the teat may help, but there are positive benefits to breast-feeding neonates with bad cleft palates since with the let-down reflex, milk is actually squirted into the mouth of the baby so that all he has to do is to swallow it. Feeding may occasionally be a persisting problem during the first few days or weeks, and periods of spoon feeding or even tube feeding may be necessary. However, this is the exception rather than the rule, and once the plate is fitted most babies nipple-feed (breast or bottle) perfectly satisfactorily.

Surgeons differ in the time at which they close the defect and there is a move to correct the lip within the neonatal period and the palate at 3 months.

CONGENITAL DISLOCATION OF THE HIP

On the basis of the examination described on pp. 101–4 hips can be classified into two groups:
- *Normal:* including clickers and creakers.
- *Abnormal:* including unstable, dislocatable, dislocated and reducible, dislocated and irreducible and ultrasonically dysplastic.

Normal hips clearly need no treatment. Although some authorities may argue for a watching brief on unstable hips, most would treat all babies in the abnormal group by using, in consultation with the local orthopaedic surgeon, one of the many splinting devices available (Fig. 20.2). The device should be put on as soon as the diagnosis is made, but great care should be taken not to immobilise the hip in full (or extreme) abduction since this may compromise the blood supply to the femoral head and cause avascular necrosis – a disaster.

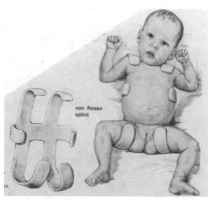

FIGURE 20.2(a) The Von Rosen splint for CDH (reproduced from Hensinger, 1979, with permission).

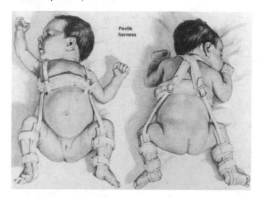

FIGURE 20.2(b) The Pavlik harness for CDH (reproduced from Hensinger, 1979, with permission).

The apparatus should stay on all the time, and the mother should be shown how to nurse her baby in it, and in particular how to change his nappy.

The fact that early diagnosis and treatment of congenital dislocation of the hip carries an excellent prognosis for an entirely normal hip joint in the future must be explained to the parents.

TALIPES

TALIPES CALCANEO-VALGUS

In this condition the back of the foot is pressed against the front of the shin (Fig. 20.3) but this is of no clinical importance, always corrects completely

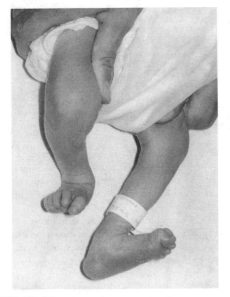

FIGURE 20.3 Talipes calcaneo-valgus.

and spontaneously, and no therapy is required. If the mother needs some occupational therapy and is anxious, she can be allowed to spend 5–10 minutes after one or two feeds per day stretching the baby's foot down towards the plantigrade position.

TALIPES EQUINO-VARUS

In this condition the foot is inverted and supinated, and adducted distal to the talus (Fig. 20.4); this is a serious malformation which needs treatment. Many babies are born with a minor degree of positional talipes equino-varus in which full ankle movements are

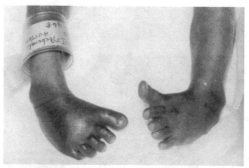

FIGURE 20.4 Talipes equino-varus.

possible. No treatment for these is indicated. However, for those with a degree of deformity that does not allow full ankle movements and particularly in those whom the foot cannot even be manipulated into a plantigrade position, early treatment is essential.

Initially treatment can be started by the neonatal staff applying zinc oxide plasters as shown in Fig 20.5. If this is started early, many feet which were not plantigrade on day one will be by two weeks of age and little if any more treatment will be needed. More severe deformities will need longer-term orthopaedic management and follow-up.

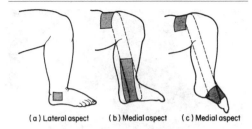

(a) Lateral aspect   (b) Medial aspect   (c) Medial aspect

FIGURE 20.5 Diagrams of strapping for talipes equinovarus. (a) shows the correct position of the leg and ankle, with both knee and ankle at a right-angle. A small square of adhesive felt protects the malleolus. (b) Shows the first length of strapping in place (viewed from the medial aspect). (c) Shows the second length of strapping in place. This second length is applied on top of the piece illustrated in (b) which has not been drawn into (c) so that the details of the later strapping can be more clearly illustrated (from Davies *et al.*, 1972, with permission).

METATARSUS VARUS

In this condition the forefoot is angled medially (Fig. 20.6) but is usually fully mobile and functional, in which case no treatment is required. If the deformity is fixed or persistent, serial plaster casts to correct the alignment of the foot may be indicated.

LIMB ABNORMALITIES

Reduction deformities of one or more limbs are rare but a cause of major, and understandable, distress in parents. Clearly, nothing can be done in the short term, but long-term orthopaedics, plastic surgery and prosthetic care will need to be planned.

It should always be remembered that some limb deformities are part of syndromes with other implications, e.g. radial clubbed hands with thrombocytopenia (TAR syndrome); absent thumbs and/or radii with congenital heart disease (Holt–Oram

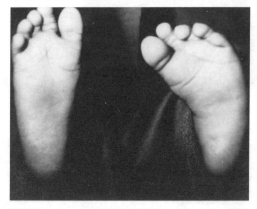

FIGURE 20.6 Metarsus varus (reproduced from Hensinger and Jones, 1992, with permission).

syndrome). The likelihood of such an association should always be checked against the catalogues.

Abnormalities of the digits are common and in general require no treatment. An extra digit on the ulnar border of the hand, a condition which is frequently dominantly inherited, is very common. Unless attached by a very narrow pedicle which can be tied off, these extra digits should be removed as a formal plastic surgery procedure.

Syndactyly between the second and the third toes is the most common malformation in Caucasians. It does not require treatment. Overlapping between the second and third toes is also common. This does not require treatment either.

AMBIGUOUS GENITALIA

Being unable to sex a newborn baby is one of the most awful catastrophes which can befall parents, and demands immediate paediatric help. Every effort must be made to establish the baby's sex within a few days, and in the meantime the parents must be kept fully in the picture about the time course of the investigations, the aims of treatment and the likely outcome; they should be discouraged from using potentially bisexual Christian names like Leslie(ey), Vivian or Franci(e)s. It is safe to nurse these babies on the PNW of a large maternity unit, but because diagnostic speed and efficiency are of the essence, and there is a risk of sudden collapse, such babies should never be kept in small, poorly equipped maternity hospitals lacking appropriate laboratory support.

The initial steps in the assessment are:

- Are testes present?; the baby is then a *male* pseudohermaphrodite.
- Can a uterus be palpated on rectal examination or demonstrated on ultrasound?; the baby is then a *female* pseudohermaphrodite.
- Could the external genitalia ever be fashioned into a sexually functional penis irrespective of the endocrine or chromosome findings?. If not, the baby should probably be reared as female.
- Is the baby hypertensive?; this localises the abnormality to the adrenal.
- Send a blood sample for urgent chromosome analysis. With modern techniques, the result may be available within 72 hours.
- Send blood and urine samples for urgent analysis to establish the diagnosis of congenital adrenal hyperplasia.

The most common diagnosis in a baby with ambiguous genitalia is that it is a girl masculinised by CAH (i.e. no testes, uterus palpable, karyotype 46XX). It is essential to remember when managing babies with ambiguous genitalia on a PNW that towards the end of the first week, or early in the second week, they may, if suffering from the salt-losing form of CAH, suddenly develop an Addisonian crisis and collapse (p. 303). To prevent this happening their plasma electrolytes should be checked daily to exclude a trend towards hyponatraemia and hyperkalaemia; urinary electrolytes should also be checked for the high urinary sodium loss which is also very characteristic of CAH. Hypertension also strongly suggests or CAH, although the salt-losing form may present with profound hypotension most commonly in the second week of life. The diagnosis of CAH is confirmed by demonstrating an elevated plasma 17-0H progestrone (21α-hydroxylayse deficiency), or 11-deoxycortisol (11-βhydroxylase deficiency), in the presence of appropriate plasma and urine electrolyte changes and/or hypertension. Once a diagnosis is established, replacement therapy should be started with steroids and salt.

If CAH is not present, or clinical and genetic examination shows that the baby is a male, more sophisticated endocrinological and gynaecological investigations will need to be carried out.

HYPOSPADIAS

The diagnosis and severity of this condition is usually obvious on examination of the baby's penis (p. 105), and so long as he can pass urine through the abnormally sited meatus, no neonatal treatment is indicated. Rarely, extreme perineo-scrotal hypospadias can give the appearance of ambiguous genitalia, but the presence of testes on examination and the absence of any biochemical defect (see above) establishes the correct diagnosis.

Repair of hypospadias is usually undertaken during the third year when the baby is dry and out of nappies.

DWARFS

Various short-limbed dwarfs (Table 20.3) may be recognised at birth or on a PNW and are healthy, but small. The lethal variants pose problems immediately after delivery and may be very difficult to resuscitate because of associated pulmonary hypoplasia. They should all be carefully assessed clinically and radiologically to establish an accurate diagnosis; this helps one to forecast the two things which concern the parents most, the baby's ultimate height, and the recurrence risk.

TABLE 20.3 Features of some skeletal dysplasias presenting at birth

Syndrome	Bony features	Outcome
Asphyxiating thoratic dystrophy (AR)	Short ribs +++ Narrow chest	Usually lethal but can survive
Achondroplasia (AD)	Short tubular bones, head large	Good
Diastrophic dwarfism (AR)	Thick, short tubular bones especially first metacarpal	Good
Camptomelic dysplasia (AR)	Bent long bones Narrow chest	Usually lethal Low IQ
Rhizomelic chondrodysplasia punctata (AR)	Short femora and humeri. Epiphyseal punctate calcification. Large head	Usually lethal Low IQ
Osteogenesis imperfecta (AR)	Multiple fractures, poorly mineralised bones	Usually lethal; survivors have multiple fractures
Osteogenesis imperfecta (AD)	Thin, fractures in early life	Multiple fractures in early life – usually wheelchair bound

AR = autosomal recessive.
AD = autosomal dominant.

MENINGOMYELOCELE

The majority of babies with open neural tube defects will be admitted to the NNICU for full neurological assessment. In general babies with one or more of:
- total paraplegia or minimal hip flexion
- kyphoscoliosis present at birth
- hydrocephalus present at birth

- a lesion > four spinal segments
- other serious malformations

will not be offered surgery in the immediate neonatal period. Such babies should have their spinal lesions dressed with a non-adhesive dressing, and be demand fed. Appropriate analgesia should be given, but sedation is usually inappropriate. Many parents of these babies will choose to care for them in the PNW or at home (see below and p. 326).

Babies with small skin-covered defects – meningoceles – do not normally require NNICU admission and can be cared for on a routine PNW. They must be carefully examined to identify minor neurological defects, e.g. slight foot weakness, or sphincter disturbances, and sinuses or other potential sites of entry for infection must be identified. A cranial ultrasound scan to exclude mild hydrocephalus is indicated.

Careful neurological and neurosurgical follow-up is required, though operative treatment is not always indicated.

CARE OF LETHAL MALFORMATIONS

A baby born with a malformation which is inevitably lethal (hypoplastic left heart, glycine encephalopathy, trisomies 13 and 18 are recent examples we have dealt with), or with a condition for which surgery was not indicated (e.g. large neural tube defects) can stay on the PNW. Many parents of these babies wish to care for them personally during terminal care, and this should always be allowed, initially in a single room on a PNW and subsequently at home. The management of each case has to be individually tailored to the medical needs of the child and the environmental support which both parents and their other children require. Clearly they will need a lot of support from the paediatricians, the nursing, midwifery and health visiting staff and their GP. In general, such babies, as always, should be demand fed at the breast or by bottle, pain should be treated with analgesics and other problems managed symptomatically; sedation of the baby on a routine basis is never indicated.

REFERENCES

Davies, P.A., Robinson, R.J. Scopes, J.W., Tizard, J.P.M., Wigglesworth, J.S. (1972). Medical care of newborn babies. Spastic International Medical Publications. Wm Heinemann Medical Books Ltd, London, p. 58.

Drostar, D., Baskieuricz, A., Irving, N., Kennell, J.H. and Klaus, M.H. (1975). The adaptation of parents to the birth of an infant with a congenital malformation: a hypothetical model. *Journal of Pediatrics* **56**, 710–716.

Hensinger, R.N. (1979). Congenital dislocation of the hip. *Ciba Clinical Symposium* **31**, 1.

Jones, K.L. (1988). *Smith's Recognisable Patterns of Human Malformations.* 4th Ed. W.B. Saunders Co, Philadelphia, London, Toronto.

FURTHER READING

Hensinger, R.N. and Jones, E.T. (1992). Orthopaedic problems in the newborn. In: *Textbook of Neonatology*, 2nd Ed. Ed. Roberton, N.R.C. Churchill Livingstone, Edinburgh, pp. 899–914.

21

DURATION OF STAY AND DISCHARGE

NORMAL BABIES

It must be remembered that for a term baby, born in good condition and with no problems manifest by 2–3 hours, hospital has nothing to offer and he can be allowed home in perfect safety. That is not to say that he and his mother are abandoned by the medical and nursing professions, merely that they can be given the appropriate and necessary care at home; after reference to this book if necessary!

SMALL BABIES

(Chapters 11 and 12)

A similar philosophy should apply to babies weighing around 2.00 kg. They can be discharged home when they are feeding satisfactorily 3 hourly, can sustain their body temperature at a room temperature of 21–22°C and the home surroundings have been checked by the health visitor or general practitioner and are known to be satisfactory. There is no need to insist on the baby reaching a predetermined body weight, and 1.60–1.80 kg neonates can, and have been discharged home in complete safety (Davies *et al.*, 1979).

BABIES WITH MALFORMATIONS

For most babies with a malformation which can be managed on a PNW such as congenital dislocation of the hip, talipes or hypospadias which is unlikely to compromise feeding, and for which no urgent therapy is required, the criteria for discharge are the same as for any other neonate of comparable gestation or birthweight. It is essential of course to have clear follow-up arrangements made before the baby is discharged.

HARELIP AND CLEFT PALATE

Babies with this problem, which is likely to make feeding more difficult (pp. 312–3), should be kept on the PNW until they are feeding adequately and gaining weight satisfactorily. After discharge, regular home visiting by the health visitor and GP, coupled with outpatient assessment is a perfectly safe and adequate mechanism of long-term care until surgical correction takes place. Remember that these babies are at particular risk from otitis media.

DOWN'S SYNDROME

The criteria for discharging these babies are no different from any other: adequate feeding and gaining weight. However, the parents should know the diagnosis, have had several talks with the paediatrician and should be in touch with the local support groups for handicapped children.

MEDICAL PROBLEMS

JAUNDICE

Anxieties occasionally arise over discharging very jaundiced breast-fed babies whose bilirubin levels exceed 250–300 µmol/l. However, a relaxed attitude should be taken. Once the bilirubin level in the plasma has plateaued or begun to come down, and so long as no other problem has been identified, it is highly unlikely that the bilirubin will rise again although it may take a long time to fall (p. 239). It also has to be remembered that kernicterus is unheard of in such infants, certainly at bilirubin levels <400 μmol/1. It is therefore entirely reasonable to let such jaundiced babies go home, but if their bilirubin is still >300 μmol/l at discharge, it is safer to see the baby as an out-patient 2–3 days later to check that he is still thriving, and that his bilirubin level is still falling.

ANAEMIA

Infants who have a neonatal haemolytic problem (p. 246), or have neonatal anaemia for any other reason (p. 276) may become profoundly anaemic very quickly after discharge, even though they are not jaundiced and have a normal haemoglobin at the end of the first week, after, if necessary, an exchange transfusion. They must, therefore, be seen 2–3 weeks after discharge to check their haemoglobin, and frequent follow-up continued until the haemoglobin is known to be rising to the normal range.

TERMINALLY ILL BABIES

Occasionally, the parents of babies who have inoperable malformations choose to have their babies die at home. This should never be discouraged, and on an individual basis appropriate help with the provision of equipment such a suction units and nasogastric tubes can be organised with continuing support from the community nursing services, the general practitioner and the hospital. In particular, it is important to have an arrangement whereby the parents can readmit their baby to the paediatric unit at any time of the day or night.

FOLLOW-UP

Too many babies are needlessly followed up after discharge from a maternity hospital, and the post-discharge care of most of the babies described in this book can be very safely left to the health visitor and the GP, and of course the parents themselves. In particular, there is no need to follow up a baby who was just pre-term or just small-for-dates.

The following conditions which are managed on a PNW should be routinely followed:

• Malformations	By the appropriate department: e.g. orthopaedic surgeons for CDH, plastic surgeons for cleft palate, hypospadias by urologists
• Heart murmur	Paediatricians or paediatric cardiologists
• Urinary tract infection	Paediatricians
• Haemolytic disease/anaemia	Paediatricians
• Trauma, fractures, Erb's palsy etc.	Paediatricians and/or Orthopaedic department

FEEDING

The special milks designed for post-discharge feeding of LBW babies should be used (pp. 129–30).

VITAMIN SUPPLEMENTS

Routine vitamin and iron supplements are not needed by term babies but should probably be given to the pre-term babies described in Chapter 11.

IMMUNISATION

All babies cared for on a PNW can have their full immunisation programme including pertussis, starting 2 to 3 months from the time of birth. If there are any contraindications to pertussis vaccine arising in the neonatal period (and that is doubtful) they are conditions such as purulent meningitis, large intracranial haemorrhage or gross CNS malformations which would not be cared for on a PNW.

REFERENCE

Davies, D.P., Haxby, V., Herbert, S. and McNeish, A.S. (1979). When should preterm babies be sent home from neonatal units? *Lancet* **i**, 914–916.

INDEX

Abdomen 16, 93, 94–5, 268, 296, 299–300

Abrasions 250–1

Abstinence syndrome 38–9, 40

Achondroplasia 321

Acidaemia, asphyxia 55, 56, 57–8, 66–7

Acidaemias, organic 292

Acylovir 26, 28, 219, 220

Addisonian crisis 303, 320

Admission routine 81

Adrenaline 62, 67, 68, 70

β-adrenergic agents 51

AIDS 230–1

Alcohol 17, 38, 43, 50

Allergies 131–3, 148

Amino acid metabolism errors 116, 240, 292

Anaemia 54, 71, 276–7, 326, 327

Anaesthetics 40, 46, 171

Analgesics 48, 159, 256

Antibiotics 294
  conjunctivitis 223
  cord care 76, 222
  gastroenteritis 225–6
  maternal therapy 19, 32, 42, 43
  pyrexia 32–3

respiratory illness 288
septicaemia 299
streptococcus 221, 294
toxoplasmosis 37, 228–9
urinary tract infection 223, 225

Anticoagulants 19, 42, 44

Anticonvulsants 21, 22, 42, 45, 256

Antihypertensives 47–8

Anus 95, 99, 222–3, 265–6, 300

Apgar score 58–9

Aplasia cutis 282

Apnoea 55–60, 66–7, 288–9, 292, 294, 296

Apt's test 264

Arthritis 33, 49, 101, 296,

Asphyxia 39, 47–8, 54–9, 66–9, 69–71

Asphyxiating thoracic dystrophy 321

Aspirin 44

Asthma 18, 41, 43, 132

Atropine 62, 68

Attachment see Bonding

Auditory screening 100

Autoimmune disorders see Immune disorders

Bag and mask ventilation 61, 64–6, 70
Barlow's sign 103–4
Bathing 64, 75, 78, 86
BCG vaccination 27
Behavioural states 96
Bell's palsy 253
Bicarbonate 62, 66, 67–8, 70, 266
Biliary atresia 240
Bilirubin 43, 232, 233
    see also Jaundice
Biochemical screening 114–18
Birth asphyxia 39, 47–8, 54–9, 66–9, 69–71
Birthmarks 284–5
Birthweights 6, 7–11
Bladder, enlarged 94, 299
Blood gases 19, 55, 56, 57–8, 60, 67
Blood glucose *see* Hypoglycaemia
Blood group incompatibility 53, 234–7, 244, 246
Blood pressure
    asphyxia 54–5
    CAH 320
    eclampsia 17, 45
    examination 92
    hypotension 23, 33, 48, 55
    maternal hypertension 19, 23, 33, 47–8
    normal values 82, 90
    pre-eclampsia 17, 23,

44, 45, 48
Blood transfusions 71, 276
    see also Exchange transfusions
Bonding 64, 75, 79–80, 147–8, 171–2
Bottle-feeding
    allergies 131–2, 132–3, 148
    cleft palate 313
    complementary feeds 137, 148, 156, 160, 163–4
    cost 135
    cot deaths 136
    cows' milk and formulae 126–8, 138
    crying babies 159–60
    curd-based formulae 129–30
    dehydration fever 165
    failure to thrive 136–7
    feed frequency 143
    feed volume 142–3, 189
    follow-on formulae 128–30, 193
    formula samples 148–9
    formula selection 141–2
    goats' milk 131–2
    hypoglycaemia 139, 165
    IDM 211, 212
    infections and 133–4

intelligence 137
jaundice 138–9
LBW babies 189, 194
maternal illness 17,
137–8
milk temperature 142
non-feeding babies
158–9
preterm babies 128,
194
psychological factors
135–6
social factors 134–5
soya milks 130–1
starting 141–2
stools 84, 124
teats 218
technique 142
toxins 136
twins 199, 201
vs breast-feeding
132–40
weight loss 138–9
wind 160–1
Bowel activity 84
Bowel sounds 93, 296,
300
Brachial plexus palsy
253–5
Bradycardia 35, 63, 68,
260
Brain *see* Central nervous
system
Branchial cysts 272–3
Breast-feeding
alcohol 38
allergies 132–3, 148
antenatal preparation
144

anti-infectious agents
121, 124–5, 133–4
artificial induction
121
breast abscess 155–6
breast engorgement
155, 157, 274
cleft palate 313
colostrum 119, 121,
124, 149
complementary feeds
137, 148, 156, 160,
163–5, 187–8, 190
contraception 49, 134
convenience 134–5
cost 135
cot deaths 136
crying babies 159–60
dehydration fever
165, 275
delivery suite 80,
147–8
environmental toxins
136
establishing 144–5,
147–8
expressed milk 17,
151, 155, 163, 187
failure to thrive
136–7, 153, 156,
162–5
feed duration 149
feed frequency 147–8,
160
feed volume 149–50
gastroenterological
symptoms 165
haematemesis 264
hypoglycaemia 139,

Breast-feeding *cont.*
    hypoglycaemia *cont.*
      151–2, 165, 187–8,
      280
    IDM 212
    intelligence 137
    jaundice 138–9, 151,
      165, 240, 243, 246,
      325–6
    large babies 205
    LBW babies 187–9,
      190
    let down reflex 120,
      146, 313
    maternal illness 17,
      25, 41–51, 137–8,
      159, 170
      asthma 18, 42–3
      cancer 24, 157
      CF 19–20
      epilepsy 20–2
      heart 18–19
      infections 25–8, 40,
      231
      lungs 19–20
      malnutrition 25
      myasthenia 30
      PKU 31
      psychiatric 31–2
      renal 33
      SLE 34–5
      thrombocytopenia
      28
      thyrotoxicosis 35–6
      vitamin deficiency
      37
    milk composition
      121–5, 138

milk production
    119–21, 125–6,
    147–50, 156–7, 164
monitoring 151–2
multiple births
    199–200, 202
night feeds 148
nipples 146, 150,
    153–5, 223
non-feeding babies
    158–9
one breast or two 149
position for 145–7
psychological factors
    135–6
smoking 41
social factors 134–5
stools 84, 124
supplementary
    feeding 164
vs bottle-feeding
    132–40
weight loss 138–9
wind 160–1
Breasts
    cancer of 24, 157
    neonatal 108, 111,
    274
    surgery 157
Breech births
    bruising 239, 250–1
    fractures 251–3
    head shape 248
    irritable babies 257–8
    NNU admission 170
    sternomastoid tumour
    273
Bromocriptine 157
Bronchiectasis 19

Bronchitis 19
Bruising 248, 250–1
Bullous impetigo 222

Caesarean section 170,
  171, 220, 250
Caffeine 44–5
CAH see Congenital
  adrenal hyperplasia
Calcium
  hypercalcaemia 30–1,
    68
  hypocalcaemia 31, 37,
    123, 258, 280
  milk and feeds 122,
    127, 129, 130, 131,
    132
  resuscitation 62, 68
  supplements 31, 280
Calories, milk and feeds
  122, 127, 129, 130,
  131, 132
Camptomelic dysplasia
  321
Cancer 23–4, 157–8
Candida (thrush) 222–3
Cannabis 40
Caput succedaneum
  248
Carbamazepine 21
Carbohydrates 122–3,
  127, 129, 130, 131
Cardiovascular system
  82
  congenital heart
    block 35
  cyanosis 290–1
  examination 90–2,
    109, 260, 261

heart failure 56, 67–9,
  291
infection signs 296
maternal disorders
  18–19, 23, 31, 47–8
murmurs 91–2, 260–2,
  291, 327
normal blood
  pressure 82, 90
normal heart rate 90
normal pulse rate 82,
  90–1
pulse abnormalities
  260
respiration 288
rubella 229
sounds 91–2
sudden collapse 303
ultrasound scan 305
Cataracts 99, 228, 309
Cavernous haeman-
  gioma 285
CDH see Congenital
  dislocation of hip
Central nervous system
  abnormal cry 257
  antenatal ultrasound
    307–8
  asphyxia 55
  brachial plexus palsy
    253–5
  delayed respiration 54
  enlarged fontanelles
    257
  epidural anaesthetic
    46
  facial nerve palsy 253
  fits 292–3, 304
  gestational age 110

Cardiovascular system
    cont.
    infection signs 297
    irritable babies 257–8
    jitteriness 258
    kernicterus 233
    maternal disorders
        20–2, 29–30, 256
    maternal illness
        effects 17, 20–1, 30,
        31, 36, 37, 38, 40
    meningomyelocoele
        305–6, 321–2
    neurological
        examination
        95–100, 109, 110
    pertussis immunisa-
        tion 327
    serious metabolic
        errors 292
    squint 259
    tone disorders 255–7
Cephalhaematomata
    108, 238, 249
Cerebral babies 257–8
Cervical cancer 23–4
Cervical cord injury 69
CF see Cystic fibrosis
CHD see Congenital
    heart disease
Chignon 249
Chlamydia infection 25,
    224
Chlormethiazole 45
Chlorothiazide 45
Choanal atresia 93
Choking attacks 288–9
Cholera 25
Chondrodysplasia
    punctata 321

Chorioretinitis 229
Choroid plexus cysts
    308
Cigarettes 17, 41
Circumcision 86, 302
Clavicle 251–2, 255
Clear fluids 142
Cleft palate 21, 93, 120,
    263, 308, 312–13,
    325
Clifford's syndrome
    182–3, 185
Clinodactyly 101, 310
CMV see
    Cytomegalovirus
Coarctation 91, 291, 305
Cocaine abuse 39
Coeliac disease 22
Colic 161–2
Colitis 22, 266
Colorectal cancer 24
Colostomy 34
Colostrum 119, 121,
    124, 149
Congenital adrenal
    hyperplasia (CAH)
    118, 303, 319–20
Congenital dislocation
    of hip (CDH) 102–4,
    313–15, 324
Congenital heart disease
    (CHD)
    cyanosis 290–1
    examination 92, 260,
        261
    IDM 213
    maternal 18, 19
    maternal PKU 31
    respiration 288

rubella 228, 229
sudden collapse 303
ultrasound 305
Congenital infections 227–31
Congenital malformations *see* Malformations; named malformations
Conjunctivitis 76, 223
Contraception 49, 134
Convulsions *see* Fits
Coombs test 34, 235
Cord
blood gas analysis 60
care 75, 85, 222
clamping 75, 302
examination 95
haemorrhage 301–2
umbilical granuloma 269
umbilical hernia 269
Cot deaths 41, 82, 136, 290
Cough 259, 296
Cows' milk and formulae 126–8
Coxsackie virus 302
Cranial nerves 99–100, 253
Craniostenosis 97
Craniosynostosis 36
Cri-du-Chat syndrome 257
Crigler–Najjar syndrome 243
Crohn's disease 22
Crying 159–60, 163, 257–8, 297

Curd-based formulae 129–30
Cutis marmorata 281
Cuts, in birth 250
Cyanosis 71, 90, 251, 290–1
Cystic dysplasia 299
Cystic fibrosis (CF) 19–20, 117–8, 300
Cystic hygromas 273, 306
Cytomegalovirus (CMV) 17, 26, 228
Cytotoxic drugs 24, 34, 42, 45

Dacrocystis 223
Deafness 43, 100, 228, 233
Dehydration 46, 165, 226, 239, 242, 275, 298
Delivery *see* Labour and delivery
Depression 31, 32
Dermal sinus 96
Dermatitis 283
Dermoid cysts 273
Dextrose 46–7, 62, 68, 160, 164, 242, 279
Diabetes, IDM 203, 204, 209–14
Diaphragmatic hernia 71, 93, 305–6
Diarrhoea 46, 226, 227, 295
Diastasis recti 108, 268, 274
Diastrophic dwarfism 321

Digits 21, 101, 274, 309, 311, 318

Discharge home 81, 193, 201, 214, 324–8

Diuretics 46

Dopamine 48, 68

Down's syndrome 97, 101, 310–12, 325

Drug addiction 17, 38–40

Duchenne muscular distrophy 118

Duodenal atresia 267, 311

Dwarfism 321

Dysmaturity 6

Dyspnoea 93, 287–8

Dystrophia myotonica 30, 256

Ears 43, 100, 111–12, 228, 233

Echovirus infection 303

Eclampsia 17, 45

Eczema 132, 219

Edrophonium 30, 257

Eisenmenger's syndrome 19

Embryo, definition 10

Endotracheal intubation 61, 64, 65, 66, 67, 70

ENT disorders 93

Eosinophil rash of newborn 282

Epidermolysis bullosa 285

Epidural anaesthetic 46, 171

Epilepsy 20–2

Epstein's pearls 108, 263

Epulis 263

Erb's palsy 100, 253, 255, 327

Ergotamine 46

Erythema 108, 230, 280–1, 282

Escherichia coli 84, 222, 224, 226, 227, 294

Examination of neonates 87–113

Exchange transfusions 33, 34, 235–6, 237, 242, 244

Exomphalos 305–6

Eyes
  cataracts 99, 228, 309
  conjunctivitis 78, 223
  delivery suite care 27, 76
  examination 99
  exophthalmos 36
  facial nerve palsy 253
  neurological assessment 110
  puffy eyelids 251
  squint 259
  subconjunctival haemorrhage 108, 251

Face 21, 101, 248, 250, 274, 281, 284

Facial nerve palsy 253, 259

Failure to thrive 136–8, 153, 156, 162–5

Fat necrosis, subcutaneous 274, 282–3

Fats, milks and feeds 123, 129, 130, 131, 138

Feeding *see* Bottle-feeding; Breast-feeding; Tube-feeding

Feet 112–13, 274, 315–16, 317–18

Femoral fractures 252–3

Fetal alcohol syndrome 38

Fetus, definition 10

Fifth disease 230

Fissure-in-ano 265–6

Fits 96, 292–3, 304
  ergotamine 46
  hypocalcaemic 31
  hypovitaminosis D 37
  infection 297
  jitteriness compared 258
  maternal 20, 21

Folic acid
  jaundice 34, 246
  milks and feeds 122, 127, 129, 130, 131

Fontanelles 97, 257, 297

Food allergies *see* Allergies; Coeliac disease

Forceps deliveries 238, 250, 253, 257–8, 282

Forearm fractures 252, 253

Foreskin 86, 105, 108, 302

Formula feeds see Bottle-feeding

Fractures 101, 251–3, 255, 327

Frusemide 62

G6PD deficiency 237, 246

Galactosaemia 117, 240

Gastroenteritis 26, 139, 219, 225–7, 267

Gastrointestinal tract
  abdominal distension 268, 299–300
  antenatal ultrasound 308
  breast-feeding 165
  common problems 263–9
  examination 94–5
  intestinal obstruction 267, 268, 300–1
  maternal disease 22
  necrotising enterocolitis 301
  stools 84, 265
  vomiting 266–8, 296

GBS 54, 221, 294

General anaesthetic 46, 171

Genital herpes 26, 220

Genitourinary tract
  abdominal distension 299–300
  Addisonian crisis 303, 319
  ambiguous genitalia 104, 303, 319–20
  bruised genitalia 250
  circumcision 86, 302
  common problems 269–72

Genitourinary tract *cont.*
  examining genitalia
    104–5
  gynaecological
    malformations
    307–8
  hypospadias 105, 271,
    320
  maternal drug
    therapy 49, 51
  maternal renal
    disorders 17, 33
  renal malformations
    306
  testicles 105, 268, 270
  urinary tract
    abnormalities 94–5
  urinary tract infection
    223, 225, 267, 327
  urine output 83–4,
    94, 271, 272
  vagina 104, 270, 271
Gestation 5–6, 7–11,
  109–12
Glabellar tap 111
Glucose
  G6PD deficiency 237,
    246
  intravenous 46–7
  see also
    Hypoglycaemia
Gluten 22, 206
Goats' milk 131–2
Goitre 35, 36, 272
Gonorrhoea 27, 224
Graves' disease 35
Group A streptococcus
  27
Group B streptococcus

  54, 221, 294
Grunting 287, 296
Guthrie tests 114, 115,
  116, 117, 118

Haemangiomas 96, 284,
  285
Haematemesis 264, 301
Haematuria 270
Haemoglobinopathies
  22–3
Haemolytic jaundice
  235, 236, 237–8, 244,
  245
Haemophilia 302
Haemophilus 224
Haemorrhage 301–2
  cord clamping 76
  haematemesis 264,
    265, 301
  haemorrhagic disease
    21, 77–8, 246, 264
  intracranial 303
  maternal thrombocy-
    topenia 29
  melaena 265, 301
  pallor with 276–7, 301
  recurrent antepartum
    17
  resuscitation 71
  subconjunctival 108,
    251
  subgaleal 250, 302
Haemorrhagic diathesis
  297
Hair 280
Hands
  abnormalities 274,
    309, 311, 317–8

examination 101
skin tags 274
washing 84, 218, 219, 220
Harelip 21, 120, 263, 308, 312, 313, 325
Harlequin colour change 281
Hayfever 132
Head
  birth injuries 248, 249, 250
  cephalhaematomata 108, 238, 249
  enlarged fontanelles 257
  examination 97
  growth abnormalities 229
  lumps on 273
  subgaleal haemorrhage 250, 302
Hearing 43, 100, 228, 233
Heart see Cardiovascular system
Heavy-for-dates see Large-for-dates
Heminevrin 45
Heparin 19, 44
Hepatitis 26, 38, 230
Hernia 105
  diaphragmatic 71, 93, 305–6
  hiatus 267
  incarcerated 160
  inguinal 268
  umbilical 269
  vomiting with 267

Heroin addiction 39
Herpes 17, 18, 26, 219–20, 302
Hiatus hernia 267
Hips, CDH 102–4, 313–15
Hirschprung's disease 268, 300, 311
Histidinaemia 117
HIV infection 38, 40, 230–1
Homecare 81
  see also Discharge home
Homocystinuria 117
HTLV infection 231
Humerus, fractures 252
Huntingdon's chorea 29
Hydrocephalus 229, 309, 322
Hydrochlorothiazide 45
Hydrocoeles 105, 108, 270
Hydrocolpos 307
Hydronephrosis 299, 306
Hydrops 71–2, 230
Hyperammonaemias 255, 292
Hypercalcaemia 30–1, 69
Hyperinsulinaemia 210
Hyperkalaemia 320
Hyperparathyroidism 30–1
Hypertension 23, 33, 47–8, 320
Hypertonia 256
Hypocalcaemia 31, 37, 123, 258, 280

Hypogammaglobulinae-
mia 216
Hypoglycaemia 277–9
adrenal hyperplasia
303
breast-fed babies 139,
151–2, 165, 187–8,
277–9
IDM 210–12, 214, 279
jittery babies 258
maternal drug
therapy 47, 50–1
monitoring 185–6
preterm babies 181,
277–9
prevention 185
SFD babies 182,
183–6, 187–8,
277–9
treatment 186,
210–12, 277–9
twins 199
Hypomagnesaemia,
IDM 213
Hyponatremia 50, 304,
320
Hypoplastic left heart
302, 322
Hypospadias 106, 271,
320, 325
Hypotension 23, 33, 48,
55
Hypothermia see
Temperature control
Hypothyroidism 36,
116, 240, 272
Hypotonia 30, 45, 51,
255–7, 292

Hypoxic ischaemic
encephalopathy 258

IDM see Infants of
diabetic mothers
Ileostomy 34
Ileus 51, 268, 300
Immaturity 6
Immune disorders
maternal 18, 28–9, 30,
34–6, 230–1
neonatal 23, 228,
256–7, 272, 283
Immunisation 22, 194,
201, 214, 231, 327
Immunoglobulins
ABO incompatibility
237–8
breast milk 121, 123,
124
cellular immunity
215–6
humoral immunity
216–17
maternal disorders 18,
26, 28, 29, 30, 33,
35
Impetigo 219
Infancy, definition 12
Infant mortality rate 15
Infants of diabetic
mothers (IDM)
209–14
Infections
breast milk 121,
124–5, 133–4
cellular immunity
215–16
congenital 227–31

cord care 77
cross infection 217–19
humoral immunity 216–7
maternal 17, 25–8, 32–3, 37, 217, 219–21
neonatal unit risks 169–70
nursing and medical staff 169–70, 217, 218, 219
physical defences 215
prevention 84–5, 217–19, 222, 230–1
serious 54, 293–9
treatable on postnatal ward 222–7
Influenza 25
Inguinal hernia 268
Intelligence 137
Intensive care 168–74, 175–6, 182, 184, 287–304
Intestinal obstruction 267, 268, 300–1
Intrauterine growth retardation (IUGR) 17, 19, 21, 33
Intubation
haematemesis with 263–4
resuscitation 61, 64, 65, 66, 70
stridor 93, 259
tracheo-oesophageal fistula 290

Intussusception 160, 266
Iodine 35, 36, 50
IPPV 45, 64, 67, 68, 70
Iron
maternal deficiency 23
milks and feeds 23, 122, 123, 124, 128, 129, 130, 131
supplements 246, 265, 276, 327
Irritable babies 45, 161–2, 257–8, 295

Jaundice 232–46
antenatal therapy 21
blood group incompatibility 235–6, 237, 244, 246
breast-fed babies 138–9, 151, 165, 239, 242, 246, 325–6
bruising 238, 250–1
causes summarised 240–1
discharge 325–6
IDM 213
induced labour 49, 239
infection marker 237–8, 295
investigation 241
kernicterus 232–3, 326
large babies 205–6
maternal epilepsy 21

Jaundice *cont.*
  NSHA 237
  physiological 238–9
  preterm babies 181
  prolonged 239–41
  rapid onset 234–7
  spherocytosis 34, 237,
    244
  treatment 34, 235–6,
    237, 242–6
Jittery babies 21, 32, 37,
  258

Kernicterus 43, 232–3,
  326
  see also Jaundice
Kidneys *see*
  Genitourinary tract;
  Renal disorders
Klumpke's paralysis 254
Kyphosis 96, 322

Labelling tags 76
Labour and delivery
  AIDS 230–1
  bathing 64, 78
  bonding 64, 79–80
  breast-feeding 80, 147
  cord care 77
  cord clamping 76
  drugs during 46–7,
    48, 49, 50–1, 171
  eye prophylaxis 76–7
  injuries 248, 249,
    250–2
  labelling tags 76
  measuring babies
    78–9
  resuscitation 53–72

  temperature control
    73–5
  vitamin K prophylaxis
    77–8
Lactaid 164
Lactation 119–21
Lactoferrin 123, 124–5
Lactose 122–3, 227
Large-for-dates 10,
  203–6, 209, 212–13
Laryngoscopes 61, 65
Larynx 93
Laxatives 48, 243
LBW *see* Low-birthweight
  babies
Length measurements
  78–9
Leprosy 26
Let down reflex 120,
  146, 313
Lethal malformations
  322–3, 326
Leukemia 17, 24, 77,
  231
Light-for-dates *see* Small-
  for-dates
Limbs 42, 101, 252–3,
  318, 321
Lipomata 274
Lithium 32, 40, 42, 50
Livebirths, defined 11
Liver, enlarged 94, 299
  see also Hepatitis;
  Jaundice
Low-birthweight babies
  6, 176, 186–93
Lungs see Respiratory
  system
Lymphadenopathy 272

Lymphocyte function 215–16
Lymphomas 24, 231

Magnesium, IDM 213–4
Magnesium sulphate 40, 51
Malaria 26
Malformations 305–23, 325, 326
  antenatal ultrasound 305
  delayed respiration 53–4
  delivery 53
  fatal types 71, 322–3, 326
  follow-up care 327
  IDM 213
  maternal illness effects 21, 25, 34–5
  resuscitation 72
  SFD babies 183–4
  teratogens 19, 21, 32, 38, 41, 42, 43, 44
  twins 196, 197, 198–9
  see also named malformations
Malnutrition 24
Maple syrup urine disease 117, 292
Mastitis 155
Maternal illness 16–37
  allergic diseases 132–3
  diabetes 203, 204, 209–14
  drug therapy 41–51, 256
  HIV infection 38, 40, 230–1
  HTLV infection 231
  infections 25–8, 32–3, 36–7, 217, 219–21, 224, 227–31
  neurological 20–2, 29–30, 256
  thyroid disease 35–6, 42, 272
Measles 26
Meckel's diverticulum 266, 302
Meconium 53, 63, 69, 78, 84, 268
Melaena 265, 301
Melanoma 24
Melanotic naevi 285
Meningitis 96, 257, 294, 297, 302, 327
Meningomyelocoele 305, 322
Metatarsus varus 317
Methylxanthines 43, 44–5
Microcephaly 31, 229
Milestones 194, 201
Milia 108, 281
Miliaria 281
Milks *see* Bottle-feeding; Breast-feeding
Mineral content, milks and feeds 122, 123, 127, 128, 129, 130, 131
Miscarriage 17
Mongolian spots 284
Moro response 100, 254

Mortality statistics 12–15
Mother-child bond
   63–4, 75, 79–80,
   147–8, 171–2
Mouth 94, 222, 223,
   262–3
Mouth-to-mouth
   resuscitation 66
Mucus extractors 61,
   230
Multiple births 53,
   196–202
Multiple sclerosis 29
Mumps 26
Murmurs 91–2, 260–2,
   327
Muscle tone see Tone
Myasthenia 30, 256
Myopathies 29, 69
Myotonic dystrophy 30,
   256

Naevi 109, 284–5
Naloxone 39, 48, 62,
   66, 68, 159
Nappy rash 283
Narcotic analgesics 48,
   159
Nasal deformity 259–60
Nasal obstruction 93
Nasogastric feeding 159,
   188, 190–3, 264
Nasogastric tubes 290
Neck lumps 272–3
Neck righting 110
Necrotising enterocolitis
   266, 301
Neonatal mortality
   13–15

Neonatal period 12
Neonatal units 168–74,
   175, 182, 183,
   287–304
Nervous system see
   Central nervous
   system
Neural tube defects
   anticonvulsants 21, 42
   fatal type 322
   lipomata 274
   maternal 29
   meningomyelocele
      305–6, 322
   urinary stream 271–2
Neuroblastoma 118, 307
Neuroglycopenia 184
Nipples 145, 150, 153–5,
   223, 281
NSAID 44, 48–9
NSHA 236, 237, 246

Occiptofrontal
   circumference 96,
   110
Omphalocoeles 269
Opiate addiction 39
Oral contraception 49,
   134
Organ transplants
   18–19, 33, 45
Orogastric feeding 192
Ortolani's sign 102–3
Osteogenesis imperfecta
   257, 321
Osteomyelitis 101, 296,
   297
Otitis media 93, 139,
   160, 267, 298

Ovarian cancer 24
Ovarian cysts 307
Oxytocin 49
see also Breast-feeding,
milk production

Pallor 70, 89, 94, 276–7,
301
Paraplegia 322
Parathyroid disorders
30–1
Parvovirus 230
Pemphigus neonatorum
222
Penis 86, 105, 108, 302
see also Hypospadias
Perinatal mortality 14
Perinatal period 12
Pertussis 22, 194, 214,
327
Petechiae 45, 94, 283–4,
297
Pethidine 48
Phenindione 44
Phenobarbitone 21, 22,
243
Phenylketonuria 31, 114
Phenytoin 21, 42
Phosphates, milks and
feeds 122, 126, 127,
128, 129, 130, 131
Phototherapy 34, 243–6
Pierre Robin syndrome
312
PKU see
Phenylketonuria
Plantar creases 113
Plethoric babies 277
Pneumomediastinum
288
Pneumonia 287, 288,
294, 296
Pneumothorax 71, 92–3,
287
Polio immunity 194, 231
Polycythaemia 213, 277
Port wine stain 284
Postconceptional age 10
Postmaturity 5, 204,
207–8
Postnatal depression 32
Potassium
adrenal hyperplasia
319
milks and feeds 122,
127, 128, 129, 130,
131
Power, assessment 98
Pre-eclampsia 17, 23, 44,
45, 48
Preterm babies 5
acute maternal illness
17
discharge home 193,
194
feeding 128, 142,
186–93, 194
follow-up care 326–7
hypoglycaemia 181,
277–8, 279
immunisation 194
intensive care 175
lanugo 280
maternal hyperten-
sion 23
milestones 194
vitamins 194, 327

Prolonged rupture of membranes 221
Propanolol 36, 47
Prostaglandin E 49
Prostaglandin synthetase inhibitors 44, 48–9, 51
Proteins
  breast milk 122, 123, 124
  formula feeds 127, 129, 130
Pseudomonas aeruginosa 20
Pseudoparalysis 101, 296
Psychiatric disorders 31–2, 49–50
Psychotropic drugs 49–50
Pulse rate 81, 82, 90–1, 260
Pustular melanosis 282
Pyelonephritis 298
Pyloric stenosis 267
Pyrexia 32–3, 275

Radioiodine 35, 36, 50
Ranulae 263
Rectum 95, 106, 265–6, 300
Regurgitation 267
Renal disorders 17, 33, 49, 51, 94, 299, 306
  see also Genitourinary tract
Respiratory distress syndrome 64, 70, 93, 213, 287

Respiratory system
  anaesthetics 46
  apnoeic attack 288–9
  cot deaths 290
  cyanosis 290–1
  dyspnoea 92, 287–8
  examination 92–3, 109
  IDM 213
  infection prevention 219
  infection signs 267, 296
  intrathoracic lesions 306
  lung malformations 71
  maternal illness 18, 19–20, 25
  narcotic analgesics 48
  nasal deformity 259–60
  normal respiration rate 82, 92
  respiratory illness 287, 288
  serious metabolic errors 292
  small babies 178
  stridor 93, 259
  tachypnoea 287
  tracheo-oesophageal fistula 290
  see also Resuscitation
Resuscitation 39, 48, 53–72, 289
Rhesus incompatibility 53, 234–5, 244, 246
Rhesus sensitisation 16

Rheumatic disorders 33, 49

Rickets 37, 123

RNCE (routine examination) 88, 106–9

Rooming-in 82, 148

Rooting reflex 142, 146

RSV 25

Rubella 17, 27, 228

Sacrococcygeal pit 96, 274–5

Salmon patch 284

Sclerema 297

Scoliosis 96, 321–2

Scrawny babies 182–3, 185

Seborrhoeic dermatitis 283

Security, labelling 76

Sedatives 49–50, 256, 258

Seizures see Fits

Septicaemia 293–8

Sexually transmitted diseases 27, 38, 77, 223, 224, 229

SFD see Small-for-dates babies

Sickle cell disease 22–3

SIDS see Cot deaths

Skeletal system 101–4, 251–3, 307, 313–18, 321

Skin
    common problems 280–5
    examination 106
    gestational age 110–11
    infections 222
    maternal problems 24, 27
    tags 274

Skull
    caput succedaneum 248
    cephalhaematomata 108, 238, 249
    enlarged fontanelles 257
    examination 96–7
    head lumps 273
    intracranial calcification 229
    moulding 248

SLE see Systemic lupus erythematosus

Sleeping position 82

Small-for-dates (SFD) babies 175–94
    assessment 182
    care of mothers 176
    causes for anxiety 183–4
    centile charts 7, 9
    discharge home 193, 194, 204
    feeding 142, 186–93
    hypoglycaemia 181, 182, 183–6, 187–8, 277–8, 279
    IDM 214
    immunisation 194
    infection prevention 181

Small-for-dates *cont.*
  intensive care
    admission 175
  jaundice 181
  jitteriness 258
  maternal illness 23,
    25
  medical care 184
  observations 178
  routine medical care
    177–8
  staffing 176–7
  temperature control
    178–80
  twins 199
  vitamin supplements
    194
  weight changes 180
Smoking 17, 41
Sodium
  hyponatremia 50,
    303, 320
  milks and feeds 20,
    122, 126, 127, 128,
    129, 130, 131
Sodium bicarbonate 62,
  66, 67–8, 70, 266
Sodium valproate 21, 42
Soya milks 130–1
Spherocytosis 33–4, 236,
  237, 244
Sphincter function 99
Spine 96, 274, 275, 284,
  297–8
Spleen examination 94
Splenectomy 28
Squint 259
Stadiometers 79
Staphylococcus 156, 219,

222, 223, 224, 294
Sternomastoid tumour
  273
Steroids 18, 34, 50
Stillbirths 11, 13, 67–9
Stomas 34
Stools 84, 264–6
'Stork bite' 108, 284
Strawberry naevi 108,
  284–5
Streptococcus 27, 54,
  221, 223, 294
Stridor 93, 259
Subconjunctival
  haemorrhage 108, 251
Subcutaneous fat
  necrosis 273, 282–3
Subgaleal haemorrhage
  250, 302
Substance abuse 17,
  38–41
Suction 61, 62, 63, 69
Sudden infant death
  syndrome see Cot
  deaths
Sweat rash 281
Syndactyly 318
Syphilis 27, 229
Systemic lupus erythe-
  matosus 34–5

T cell function 215–16
Tachycardia 36, 51, 68,
  260, 296, 301
Tachypnoea 93, 287–8,
  294, 296, 301
Talipes 108, 315–16
TB 27, 43
Teeth 43, 94, 263

Temperature control
  bathing 64, 78
  delivery suite 74–5
  postnatal ward 83
  pyrexial babies 275
  resuscitation 61, 62–3
  small babies 178–80
Temperature measure-
  ment 81, 106, 295
Tendon reflexes 99
Tensilon test 30, 257
Teratogens 19, 21, 32,
  36–8, 41, 42, 43, 44
Term babies 5
Terminal care 322–3,
  326
Testicles 105, 268,
  270–1
Thalassaemia 22–3
Thrombocytopenia 23,
  28–9, 45, 229, 283
Thrush 222–3
Thyroid disease 24,
  35–6, 42, 115, 240,
  272
Tobacco smoking 17, 41
Tocolytics 50–1
Tone 30, 97–8, 255–7,
  292
Tongue 108, 262
Toxic epidermal
  necrolysis 222
Toxoplasmosis 17, 27,
  37, 228–9
Tracheo-oesophageal
  fistula 142, 290
Traction response 110
Transient tachypnoea of
  newborn 287

Traumatic cyanosis 251,
  290–1
Tridione 21, 42
Triplets 201–2
Tropical diseases 27
Tube-feeding 159, 188,
  190–3
Tuberculosis 27, 43
Twins 53, 176–7,
  196–202
Typhoid 25

Ulcerative colitis 22
Ultrasound screening
  104, 257, 305, 307–8
Umbilicus see Cord
Ureaplasma colonisation
  27
Ureterostomy 34
Urinary tract see
  Genitourinary tract

Vagina 104, 270, 271
Valproate 21, 42
Varicella virus 17, 27–8
Ventilation 64–6, 66–7,
  69–71
Ventouse deliveries 249
Very-low-birthweight 6
Vestibular system 99–100
Viability 10–11
Vision see Eyes
Visitors 85, 217
Vitamin A 42, 122, 127,
  128, 129, 130, 131
Vitamin D
  breast milk 37, 122,
    123, 138

Vitamin D *cont.*
  deficiency 31, 37, 122, 123–4
  feeds and milks 127, 129, 130, 131, 132
Vitamin E 122, 127, 129, 130, 131
Vitamin K 44, 63, 77–8, 264, 265, 302
Vitamin supplements 37, 194, 327
Vomiting 46, 142, 226, 263–4, 266–8, 295, 296

Warfarin 19, 42, 44
Weaning 206
Weight changes
  feeding 137, 138–9, 152, 156, 162–5, 190
  IDM 213
  infection 295
  large babies 205
  postnatal care 83
  test weighing 153
  twins 200
Werdnig–Hoffman disease 100, 256
Wharton's jelly 75, 77, 269
Wheat 22, 206
Whey-based milks 127–8
Wilm's tumour 24
Wilson's disease 29
Wind 160–1
Withdrawal syndrome 38–9, 40

Xiphisternum 108, 274